Student ...

to accompany

Calculating Drug Dosages:
An Interactive Approach
to Learning Nursing Math

Sandra Luz Martinez de Castillo, RN, MA

Nursing Instructor
Contra Costa College
San Pablo, California

and

Maryanne Werner-McCullough, RN, MS, MNP

Nursing Instructor
Contra Costa College
San Pablo, California

F. A Davis Company • Philadelphia

F. A. Davis Company
1915 Arch Street
Philadelphia, PA 19103
www.fadavis.com

ISBN: 0-8036-1034-3

Printed in the United States of America

Last digit indicates print number: 10 9 8 7

NOTE: Author and publisher have done everything possible to ensure content herein is accurate, current, and in accord with accepted standards at the time of publication and to secure permission to reproduce drug labels. The reader is advised that information related to drugs, including facsimiles of drug labels, is presented for demonstration purposes only to illustrate calculation methods. The reader is further advised to refer to current pharmaceutical references for information about drug therapy and always to check product information (package inserts) for new information regarding dose and contraindications before administering any drug. Caution is especially urged when using new or infrequently ordered drugs.

A Note to the Student

Dear Student:

Learning nursing math is a challenging goal. For some, math is logical and easy. For others, the mention of math brings anxiety. The CD-ROM and Student Workbook are designed to make learning nursing math fun and easy.

In the CD-ROM you will find 12 modules. Each module is developed to address the most common math concepts used in nursing practice. Within each module you will find:

- A tutorial of each math concept
- Critical thinking word problems
- Interactive learning activities
- Practice problems to help you apply the math concepts
- A choice of method (dimensional analysis, formula method, linear ratio and proportion, and fractional ratio and proportion) for solving problems
- Feedback on how to solve problems
- Section quizzes at the end of each math concept
- A module review covering all the math concepts presented in the module with answers
- Two module tests that allow you to print out your score after the completion of the test

In all the years that we have been teaching drug dosage calculations to nursing students, we always are asked for more worksheets and more practice problems. We, therefore, have designed this Student Workbook to give you extra practice with the math concepts you are learning. The Student Workbook will give you additional problems, and answers are provided in the back of the book.

Enjoy using the CD-ROM and the Student Workbook to learn, practice, and calculate drug dosages safely for your nursing practice.

We wish you success, and remember practice makes perfect!

Sandra and Maryanne

Contents

Modules

Module: BASIC MATH REVIEW

FRACTIONS

KEY POINTS:
- Check the denominators before adding and subtracting fractions. If they are different, find the lowest common denominator, then solve the problem.
- For multiplication of fractions, just multiply the numerators and the denominators.
- For division of fractions, remember to invert the second fraction. Then multiply the numerators and the denominators.
- Change all mixed numbers to improper fractions before working out the problem.
- Reduce all fractions to their lowest terms.

Working with Addition of Fractions
Add the following fractions and mixed numbers.

1. 2/5 + 1/5   = _____

2. 2/21 + 18/42   = _____

3. 2/5 + 2/3   = _____

4. 4 4/8 + 3/4   = _____

5. 2 3/4 + 1/5 + 2 1/2 = _____

6. 3 1/8 + 4 5/6 + 7 1/4 = _____

7. 8 2/9 + 2 1/5 + 3 2/3 = _____

8. $6\ 7/15 + 3\ 4/5 + 4\ 5/6$ = _____

9. $3\ 1/10 + 5\ 2/5 + 9\ 1/8$ = _____

10. $11\ 1/8 + 7\ 3/4 + 2\ 7/8$ = _____

Working with Subtraction of Fractions
Subtract the following fractions and mixed numbers.

1. $5/6 \quad - \quad 1/3$ = _____

2. $8/10 \quad - \quad 1/2$ = _____

3. $7/8 \quad - \quad 2/3$ = _____

4. $4\ 1/4 \quad - \quad 1\ 3/8$ = _____

5. $10\ 1/2 \quad - \quad 3\ 1/5$ = _____

6. $8\ 1/6 \quad - \quad 5\ 2/3$ = _____

7. $11\ 2/5 \quad - \quad 6\ 7/8$ = _____

8. $20\ 1/8 \quad - \quad 9\ 2/3$ = _____

9. $15\ 2/7 \quad - \quad 4\ 5/6$ = _____

10. $10\ 1/2 \quad - \quad 3\ 2/5$ = _____

Working with Multiplication of Fractions
Multiply the following fractions and mixed numbers.

1. 6/8   x   2/5   = _____

2. 10/9   x   1/2   = _____

3. 5/12   x   1 1/5   = _____

4. 3 1/8   x   3/10   = _____

5. 5 1/2   x   3 3/5   = _____

6. 3 1/3   x   4 3/7   = _____

7. 2 5/6   x   1 1/8   = _____

8. 4 5/7   x   2 2/5   = _____

9. 6 1/8   x   3 2/3   = _____

10. 1 1/9   x   2 11/12   = _____

Working with Division of Fractions
Divide the following fractions and mixed numbers.

1. 7/10   ÷   1/2   = _____

2. 1/150   ÷   1/3   = _____

3. 6/8   ÷   3/5   = _____

4. 4 5/7   ÷   1/2   = _____

5. 3 1/2   ÷   3 3/4   = _____

6.   2 2/5 ÷ 5 4/5   = _____

7.   4 1/8 ÷ 7 1/2   = _____

8.   6 2/9 ÷ 3 1/3   = _____

9.   4 5/7 ÷ 1/7   = _____

10. 5 1/2 ÷ 8 3/4   = _____

Decimals

DECIMALS

KEY POINTS:
- When adding and subtracting decimals, make sure that the decimal points are lined up correctly.
- For multiplication of decimals, count the total number of decimal places in the numbers multiplied. Then count the same number of decimal places in the answer and place the decimal point.
- When dividing decimals, if there is a decimal point in the divisor, move the decimal point to make the divisor a whole number. Then move the decimal point in the dividend the same number of decimal places. Place the decimal point in the answer in the same place as in the dividend.

Working with Addition of Decimals
Add the following decimals.

1.   3.7 + 5998 + 0.0032 + 72.91   = _____

2. $78.2 + 55 + 9.005$ = _____

3. $1.75 + 0.234 + 0.004$ = _____

4. $0.17 + 7 + 1954 + 0.0013$ = _____

5. $2.29 + 5.01 + 45 + 4.67$ = _____

6. $53.1 + 8.2 + 9.5$ = _____

7. $11.6 + 10 + 0.02$ = _____

8. $2.17 + 7.1 + 50 + 0.25$ = _____

9. $20.4 + 0.1 + 37 + 8.21$ = _____

10. $3.09 + 6.70 + 5 + 14.2$ = _____

11. $31.4 + 2.1 + 1.09 + 1.4$ = _____

12. $0.07 + 4.25 + 19 + 4.8$ = _____

Working with Subtraction of Decimals
Subtract the following decimals.

1. $321.02 - 0.0045$ = _____

2. $1.031 - 0.98$ = _____

3. $9012.4 - 0.067$ = _____

4. $7050.3 - 1.037$ = _____

5. $8 - 0.023$ = _____

6.   605.1 — 4.05   = _____

7.   425.2 — 1.503   = _____

8.   67.09 — 0.29   = _____

9.   9167.3 — 463.5   = _____

10.   876 — 22.9   = _____

11.   1256.3 — 702.4   = _____

12.   950 — 10.8   = _____

Working with Multiplication of Decimals
Multiply the following decimals.

1.   301.12 x 0.25   = _____

2.   2.021 x 0.8   = _____

3.   502.6 x 0.67   = _____

4.   75.3 x 1.037   = _____

5.   5.1 x 0.02   = _____

6.   201.01 x 0.15   = _____

7.   61.48 x 0.06   = _____

8.   30.6 x 0.24   = _____

9.   150 x 2.134   = _____

10.   8.25   x   0.03   = _____

11.   65.02   x   1.04   = _____

12.   10.3   x   4.9   = _____

Working with Division of Decimals
Divide the following decimals.

1.   0.9   ÷   0.02   = _____

2.   16.80   ÷   0.15   = _____

3.   382.32   ÷   54   = _____

4.   75.85   ÷   3.7   = _____

5.   0.0015   ÷   0.03   = _____

6.   100.3   ÷   0.25   = _____

7.   250.12   ÷   5.2   = _____

8.   1000.8   ÷   12   = _____

9.   70.05   ÷   1.5   = _____

10.   0.0226   ÷   0.4   = _____

11.   618.2   ÷   12.5   = _____

12.   0.542   ÷   0.5   = _____

ROMAN NUMERALS

KEY POINTS:
- Read Roman numerals from left to right.
- Remember the following rules:
    - The Roman numerals I, X, C, and M may be repeated in sequence, but only up to three times.
    - The Roman numerals V, L, and D may never be repeated.
    - A smaller numeral to the right of a larger numeral is added to the larger numeral.
    - A smaller numeral to the left of a larger numeral is subtracted from the larger numeral.

Working with Roman Numerals
Write the Roman numerals for the following arabic numbers.

1. 7 1/2   = _____

2. 35   = _____

3. 41   = _____

4. 65   = _____

5. 101   = _____

6. 15 1/2   = _____

7. 99   = _____

8. 2005   = _____

Write the Arabic numbers for the following Roman numerals.

1. **XXX** = _____

2. **XIV** = _____

3. **XLIX** = _____

4. **ISS** = _____

5. **CL** = _____

6. **XCV** = _____

7. **LXXV** = _____

8. **MMX** = _____

Module: METHODS OF CALCULATION

SELECT A METHOD
OF CALCULATION

Linear Ratio and Proportion:
5 mg : 1 tab :: 10 mg : x tab

Fractional Ratio and Proportion:

$$\frac{5 \text{ mg}}{1 \text{ tab}} = \frac{10 \text{ mg}}{x \text{ tab}}$$

Dimensional Analysis:

$$\frac{10 \text{ mg}}{1} \times \frac{1 \text{ tab}}{5 \text{ mg}} = x \text{ tab}$$

Formula:

$$\frac{10 \text{ mg}}{5 \text{ mg}} \times 1 \text{ tab} = x \text{ tab}$$

KEY POINTS:
- Learn the method of your choice: study the set-up.
- To arrive at the correct answer, the units of measurement must be set up so that they cancel.

Working with a Method of Calculation
Solve the following problems using the method of your choice.

1. The order is for 50 mg. The pharmacy sends 25 mg tablets. How many tablets will the nurse give?

   _____

2. The order is for 75 mg. The pharmacy sends 50 mg scored tablets. How many tablets will the nurse give?

   _____

3. The order is for 1 mcg. The pharmacy sends 0.5 mcg pills. How many pills will the nurse give?

_____

4. The order is for 10 gr. The pharmacy sends 40 gr scored tablets. How many tablets will the nurse give?

_____

5. The order is for 1.2 g. The pharmacy sends 0.4 g caplets. How many caplets will the nurse give?

_____

6. The order is for 7 mg. The pharmacy sends an elixir labeled 2 mg/mL. How many mL will the nurse give?

_____

7. The order is for 1 ½ gr. The pharmacy sends 0.5 gr tablets. How many tablets will the nurse give?

_____

8. The doctor orders Lanoxin 125 mcg q.d. The nurse finds the following in the patient's medication drawer. How many mL of Lanoxin will the nurse administer?

Lanoxin
500 mcg per 2 mL

_____

9. The order is for IV ranitidine 75 mg q.8h. The pharmacy sends the following vial of ranitidine. How many mL will the nurse give?

> **Ranitidine for Injection**
>
> **25 mg/mL**

_____

10. The order is for 100 mg. The pharmacy sends a suspension labeled 12.5 mg/2 mL. How many mL will the nurse give?

_____

11. The order is for amoxicillin/clavulanate 250 mg t.i.d. The pharmacy sends the following medication. How many days will the bottle last?

> Amoxicillin/Clavulanate
> Potassium Tablets
>
> 250 mg / tablet
>
> **Contains 30 tablets.**

_____

12. The order is for 125 mg b.i.d. The pharmacy sends a 200 mL bottle labeled 12.5 mg/mL. How many days will the bottle last?

_____

13. The order is for 0.015 g of medication IM stat. The pharmacy sends a vial of the medication labeled 0.01 g per 1.5 mL. How many mL will the nurse administer?

_____

14. The physician orders 21 mg p.o. t.i.d. The nurse has a 100 mL bottle labeled 6 mg/mL. How much will the patient receive?

_____

15. The patient is to receive 60 mcg p.o. q.d. The nurse has a bottle labeled 4 mcg/2 cc. How much will the patient receive each day?

_____

16. The physician orders heparin sodium 6000 U SC q.12h. The pharmacy sends the following vial of heparin. How many mL will the patient receive per dose?

> **Heparin Sodium**
> **10,000 U/mL**

_____

17. The doctor orders gr 1/150 b.i.d. The pharmacy sends a bottle labeled gr 1/150 per pill.   How many gr will the patient receive each day?

_____

18. The patient has an order for amoxicillin oral suspension 500 mg q.8h. The medication drawer contains the following bottle of amoxicillin. How many mL will the patient receive per dose?

> # Amoxicillin Oral Suspension
>
> ### 125 mg in 5 mL
>
> For oral use only. Shake well before use.

_____

19.a. The doctor orders 0.4 mg of a medication b.i.d. The pharmacy sends a vial labeled 1 mg/mL. How many mL will the patient receive?

_____

b. If the vial contains 2 mL, how many doses are contained in the vial?

_____

20.a. The order is for heparin 8000 U SC now. The pharmacy sends the following dose of heparin. Calculate the number of mL the patient will receive.

> **Heparin Sodium**
>
> 10,000 U/mL
>
> Multidose vial containing 4 mL

_____

b. How many doses will the nurse be able to give from the above vial?

_____

c. If the order is changed to heparin 6500 U SC daily, how many mL will the patient receive per dose?

_____

d. How many doses of the above order would the nurse be able to give from the vial?

_____

Module: SYSTEMS OF MEASUREMENT

METRIC SYSTEM:
UNITS OF MEASUREMENT

Kilo Hecto Deka BASIC Deci Centi Milli Micro
UNIT

KEY POINTS:
- Memorize the metric units of measurement, metric abbreviations, and the metric line.

Working with the Metric System
Fill in the blanks with the correct answer.

1.   3.500 L = _____ mL

2.   0.7 L = _____ mL

3.   1000 mg = _____ g

4.   100 mcg = _____ mg

5.   10 mg = _____ mcg

6.   2 mg = _____ mcg

7.   35.6 mg = _____ g

8.   7.45 mL = _____ L

9.   0.07 cm = _____ dm

10.   10 km   = _____ M

11.   100 cm   = _____ mm

12.   1.65 kg = _____ g

13.   1500 mL = _____ L

14.   2.5 g = _____ mg

15.   The patient receives vancomycin 750 mg IV b.i.d. How many g does the patient receive per dose?

       _____

16.   The patient has an order for 0.5 g of ampicillin. How many mg will the nurse administer?

       _____

17.   The patient receives levothyroxine 75 mcg p.o. q.d. How many mg does the patient receive?

       _____

18.   The doctor's order is for Lanoxin elixir 0.45 mg p.o. This dose is equivalent to _____ mcg.

       _____

19.   The weight of a medication is 1.2 kg. This is equivalent to __ g.

       _____

20.   A wound measures 4 cm in length. This is equivalent to _____ mm.

       _____

APOTHECARIES' SYSTEM: UNITS OF MEASUREMENT

UNIT	ABBREVIATION	SYMBOL
grain	gr	--
minim	m	ℳ
dram	dr	ʒ
ounce	oz	ʒ

KEY POINTS:
- Memorize the units of measurement, abbreviations, and symbols used in the apothecaries' system.
- Review the rules of Roman numerals.

Working with the Apothecaries' System
Fill in the blanks using Roman numerals and symbols.

1.   3 drams = _____

2.   10 minims = _____

3.   8 ounces = _____

4.   14 minims = _____

5.   7 ½ grains = _____

6.   34 grains = _____

7.   ½ dram = _____

8.   19 ounces = _____

9. The nurse is charting 4 ounces of medication on the medication record. Use the symbol and Roman numeral to write 4 ounces.

_____

10. Write 12 minims using the correct symbol and Roman numerals.

_____

11. The nurse gives 1 ounce of antacid to the patient. Fill in the medicine cup below.

```
        —    1 FL OZ   —
         —  3/4 FL OZ  —
          — 1/2 FL OZ —
          — 1/4 FL OZ —
           — 1/8 FL OZ —
```

12. The nurse gives 1 dram of cough syrup to the patient. Fill in the medicine cup below.

```
          —  8 DRAMS  —
          —  6 DRAMS  —
          —  4 DRAMS  —
          —  2 DRAMS  —
           —  1 DRAM  —
```

HOUSEHOLD SYSTEM:
UNITS OF MEASUREMENT

UNIT	EQUIVALENT MEASUREMENT	ABBREVIATION
1 glass	8 ounces	--
1 cup	8 ounces	--
1 teacup	6 ounces	--
1 tablespoon	3 teaspoons	T, Tbs
1 teaspoon	5 mL	t, tsp
1 drop	1 minim	gt
2.2 pounds	1 kilogram	lb

KEY POINTS:
- Memorize the units of measurement, equivalent measurements, and symbols used in the household system.

Working with the Household System
Fill in the blanks with the correct answer.

1.   Two Tbs   = _____ tsp

2.   One ounce   = _____ T

3.   One-half ounce   = _____ tsp

4.   Two glasses of juice   = _____ oz

5.   One cup   = _____ oz

6.   ℈i   = _____ t

7. Three tsp of an antacid   = _____ T
Fill in the medicine cup below.

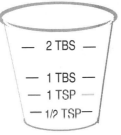

8. The nurse administers 2 tsp of cough syrup to the patient. How many mL will the nurse administer?

_____

Fill in the medicine cup below.

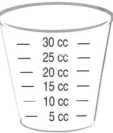

9. The patient drinks 3 glasses of water. How many ounces did the patient drink?

_____

10. The nurse gives the patient a cup of broth. How many ounces is this?

_____

CONVERSIONS BETWEEN SYSTEMS: UNITS OF MEASUREMENT

UNIT		EQUIVALENT MEASUREMENTS	
1 inch	=	2.54 cm	
60 mg	=	1 gr	
15 gr	=	1 g	
1 oz	=	30 mL	= 2 T
1 dr	=	4 mL	
1 tsp	=	5 mL	
1 T	=	15 mL	= 3 tsp
1 glass	=	8 ounces	= 240 cc
1 cup	=	8 ounces	= 240 cc
1 teacup	=	6 ounces	= 180 cc
1 gt	=	1 minim	
16 minims	=	1 mL	
2.2 lb	=	1 kilogram	

KEY POINTS:

- Memorize the equivalent measurements for each of the three systems of measurement: metric, apothecaries', and household.

Working with Conversions between Systems
Fill in the blanks with the correct answer.

1. 1/2 oz = ____mL   6. gr ss = ____mg

2. gr 1/150 = ____mg   7. 45 mL = ℥ ____

3. 2 T = ____oz   8. 12 mL = ℥ ____

4. 0.3 mg = gr____   9. gr 1/100 = ____mg

5. gr iii = ____mg   10. ℳ iv = gtt____

11.   20 mL = ____ t   15. 1 g   = gr ____

12.   3 T = ____ t   16. 75 kg = ____ lb

13.   2 cups = ____ cc   17. 198 lb = ____ kg

14.   1 inch = ____ cm   18. ℥ XLViii = ____ cc

19.   The doctor order thyroid gr ¼ p.o. for the
       patient. Thyroid is available in 30 mg tablets.
       How many tablets will the nurse give?

       _____

20.   The patient drinks two 6 oz cups of coffee for
       breakfast. How many cc did the patient drink?

       _____

21.   A patient weighs 84 kg. How many pounds does
       the patient weigh?

       _____

22.   Order: cephalexin gr viiss
       Available: cephalexin 0.250 g per tablet

       How many tablets will the nurse give?

       _____

23.   The physician orders morphine sulfate 5 mg IV
       for the patient. The narcotic drawer contains
       ampules of morphine sulfate labeled 15 mg/mL.
       How many mL will the nurse administer?

       _____

Module: INTAKE AND OUTPUT

INTAKE AND OUTPUT:
EQUIVALENT MEASUREMENTS

1 glass	8 ounces	240 cc
1 cup	8 ounces	240 cc
1 teacup	6 ounces	180 cc
1 styrofoam cup	6 ounces	180 cc
1 Popsicle	3 ounces	90 cc

ice cubes   (melt to ½ the original volume)

1 ounce (oz)	30 cc
1 dram (dr)	4 cc
1 tablespoon (T, Tbs)	15 cc
1 teaspoon (t, tsp)	5 cc

KEY POINTS:
- Intake and output (I & O) is calculated in cc.
- The size of food containers varies, so it is important for the nurse to become familiar with the specific containers used in each clinical setting.
- Parenteral intake is calculated as a part of the total intake.

Working with Intake and Output
Add the following intakes and outputs.

1. The patient is on strict I & O. For breakfast the patient took 1 cup of coffee, a 4 ounce glass of juice, and 240 mL of milk. For lunch the patient had a styrofoam cup of tea and 6 ounces of broth. The patient voided 260 mL at 1000, and 180 mL at 1400. Calculate the patient's I & O.

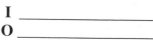

I _____

O _____

2. The patient is n.p.o. for breakfast. For lunch the patient was allowed to take 120 mL of water. The patient vomited 180 cc at 1300 and voided 100 mL at 1330. At 1400 the patient took 2 T of jello and ½ glass of apple juice. Calculate the patient's I & O.

I _____

O _____

3. The patient has a NG tube connected to low wall suction. At 0930 the M.D. wrote an order to clamp the NG tube. The nurse emptied 280 cc of NG drainage. At 1100 the patient vomited 325 cc of bile-colored drainage. The NG tube was reconnected to suction and drained an additional 475 cc by the end of the shift. The patient's wound drainage tube collected 60 cc of serosanguineous fluid. The patient's indwelling urinary catheter drained 270 cc of dark amber urine. Calculate the patient's output.

O _____

4. A patient who had prostate surgery yesterday has an indwelling urinary catheter with continuous bladder irrigation. He is n.p.o. for breakfast and is started on a clear liquid diet for lunch. He took 6 ounces of broth and 4 ounces of cranberry juice. By the end of the shift, the nurse calculates that 2000 cc of bladder irrigant has infused. The total amount emptied from the urinary bag was 2270 cc. Calculate the I & O.

I _____

O _____

5.   The patient has an IV of D5W infusing at 125 cc/hr. For breakfast the patient took 1 glass of juice and a cup of coffee. For lunch the patient took six ounces of soup and a 12 ounce can of soda. The patient voided 220 cc at 1000 and 375 cc at 1400. Calculate the patient's 8 hr total I & O.

I _____

O _____

6.   At 0700, the patient is n.p.o. and has a primary IV of 1 L of D5NS q.10h infusing continuously. The patient receives gentamicin 80 mg IVPB in 100 cc NS at 0900–1700–0100 and metronidazole 500 mg in 100 cc NS at 0800. Calculate the patient's total parenteral intake starting at 0700 and ending at 1500.

I _____

7.   At 0700, the nurse started an IV of 1 L LR and set the infusion pump at 83 mL/hr. The patient was put on strict I & O. The patient was started on cimetidine 300 mg IVPB in 50 cc NS at 0800–1400–2000–0200. For breakfast, the patient took 1 cup of coffee and a 6 ounce bowl of cream of wheat. He was n.p.o. except for ice chips for the rest of the shift. The patient took 6 ounces of ice chips and voided 425 cc. Calculate the patient's total I & O starting at 0700 and ending at 1500.

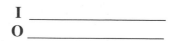

I _____

O _____

26

8. At 1500 the patient had an IV of 1 L of D5W
    infusing at 125 cc/hr. For dinner, the patient
    took 1 glass of juice and an 8 ounce can of
    nutritional supplement. The IV infiltrated at
    1800 and was restarted at 2000. The patient
    received KCl 20 mEq IVPB in 100 cc D5W at
    1700. The patient voided twice for the entire
    shift (315 cc and 290 cc). Calculate the patient's
    total I & O starting at 1500 and ending at 2300.

                    I _____
                    O _____

9. At 2300 the patient had an IV of 1 L of 0.45%
    NS infusing at 50 cc/hr. The patient had coffee-
    ground emesis measuring 480 cc at 0100. The
    M.D. ordered 2 U of PRBCs over 3 hours,
    followed by an IV of 0.9% NS to infuse at 150
    cc/hr. The nurse discontinued the current IV
    and started the first unit of PRBC (250 cc) at
    0200 and the second unit (270 cc) at 0330. The
    IV of 0.9% NS was started at 0500. Calculate
    the patient's total I & O starting at 2300 and
    ending at 0700.

                    I _____
                    O _____

10. At 1500 the patient had 900 cc left in the IV bag.
    The IV was infusing at 75 cc/hr. At 1900, the IV
    infiltrated and was restarted 1 hour later. The
    physician increased the IV rate to 125 cc/hr at
    2000. Calculate the patient's total parenteral
    intake starting at 1500 and ending at 2300.

                    I _____

NASOGASTRIC TUBE FEEDING PROBLEMS

KEY POINTS:
- Preparing dilute tube feedings requires calculating the number of mL of water to add to the tube feeding formula.
- Information needed to solve the problem includes the amount of formula in the tube feeding can and the strength of the ordered solution.

Working with Nasogastric Tube Feeding Problems

1. The doctor orders a ¾-strength tube feeding for the patient. The prepared formula comes in cans containing 240 mL. How much water will the nurse add to the can of formula to make a ¾-strength solution?

   _____

2. The patient receives a 1/3-strength tube feeding. The tube feeding can contains 233 cc. How much water will the nurse add to the can to make a 1/3-strength solution?

   _____

3. The order is to prepare a 2/3-strength tube feeding of Nepro for the patient with a percutaneous endoscopic gastrostomy (PEG) tube. How much water will the nurse add to the 237 mL can of Nepro to make a 2/3-strength solution?

   _____

4. The physician orders 200 cc of a 1/4-strength tube feeding q.6h. for a patient with a NG tube. The tube feeding can contains 250 cc. How much water will the nurse add to the can of tube feeding to make a 1/4-strength solution?

_____

5. A patient who has been receiving full-strength Jevity Plus PEG tube feedings develops diarrhea. The physician orders a diluted tube feeding of 1/2-strength Jevity Plus for the patient. How much water will the nurse add to the 237 mL can of Jevity Plus to make a 1/2 strength solution?

_____

6. The physician orders a 1/4-strength tube feeding of Osmolite at 40 cc/hr for a patient with a NG tube. The Osmolite can contains 237 mL. How much water will the nurse add to the Osmolite to make a 1/4-strength solution?

_____

7. A patient has an order for 1/2-strength Pulmocare tube feedings at 50 mL/hr through a PEG tube. The nurse prepares the dilute solution and has a total volume of 475 mL. According to hospital policy, only 4 hours of tube feeding formula can be hung at a time to prevent bacterial growth. How many mL of the prepared 1/2-strength formula will the nurse use?

_____

Module: READING MEDICATION LABELS

READING MEDICATION LABELS

KEY POINTS:

- The essential information found on medication labels includes the following:
  - trade name
  - generic name
  - dosage strength
  - form of the drug
  - route of administration
  - expiration date
  - instructions for mixing
  - recommended dose

- The useful information found on medication labels includes the following:
  - total quantity
  - manufacturer's name
  - storage information
  - lot number
  - controlled substance symbol

Working with Reading Medication Labels
Use the medication labels to fill in the answers.

1.

Rx only

See package Insert for complete product information.
Dispense in tight, light-resistant container.

Store at 25°C (77°F); excursions permitted to 15°-30°C (59°-86°F) [see USP Controlled Room Temperature].

Pramipexole was jointly developed by Pharmacia & Upjohn Company and Boehringer Ingelheim.
U.S. Pat. Nos. 4,886,812 and 4,843,086

816 997 102

Pharmacia & Upjohn Co.
Kalamazoo, MI 49001, USA

NDC 0009-0004-02

Mirapex ®
pramipexole dihydrochloride tablets

0.25 mg

90 Tablets

0009-0004-02 6

ZM3

Lot
Exp

a. Trade name _____

b. Generic name _____

c. Dosage strength _____

d. Form of the drug _____

e. Route of administration _____

2.

5 mL   SINGLE DOSE Ampul
FENTANYL
CITRATE INJ., USP   CII
250 mcg / 5 mL
50 mcg/mL (0.05 mg/mL)
Warning: May be habit forming.
For IV or IM use. Each mL con-
tains fentanyl citrate equivalent to
50 mcg (0.05 mg) fentanyl base
in Water for Injection.
PROTECT FROM LIGHT. A-1117d
ESI   ELKINS-SINN, INC.
Cherry Hill, NJ 08003

LOT

EXP.

a. Generic name _____

b. Dosage strength _____

c. Form of the drug _____

d. Routes of administration _____

e. Controlled substance?   yes_____   no_____

e. Multidose _____   Single dose_____

g. Ordered: 150 mcg IV.
    The nurse will give_____

3.

851620   NDC 0026-8562-20

Batch:
Expires:
PL500009
4759
© 1995 Bayer Corporation
Printed in USA
Store between 41-86°F (5-30°C).
Protect from light.
Avoid freezing.

CIPRO® I.V.
(ciprofloxacin)
SINGLE DOSE VIAL contains:
20 mL sterile 1% solution
200 mg **ciprofloxacin**
DILUTE BEFORE USE. For
Intravenous (iv) Infusion
Caution: Federal (USA) law
prohibits dispensing without
prescription.

FOR ADMINISTRATION, DILUTE
with 100 to 200 mL's of suitable diluent.
For complete product information,
including Dosage and Administration,
see accompanying package insert.
INACTIVE INGREDIENTS: Lactic
acid as solubilizes, HCl to adjust pH
and Water for Injection,USP.

Bayer Corporation
Pharmaceutical Division
400 Morgan Lane
West Haven, CT 06516

Bayer

a. Trade name _____

b. Generic name _____

c. Instructions for mixing _____

4.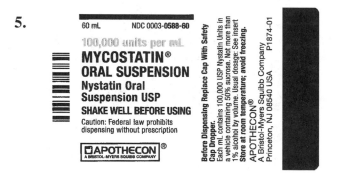

Label details:

20 mL Multiple Dose Vial
NDC 0641-2345-41
MORPHINE CII
SULFATE INJECTION, USP
15 mg/mL WARNING: May be habit forming.
FOR SUBCUTANEOUS, INTRAMUSCULAR
OR SLOW INTRAVENOUS USE
NOT FOR EPIDURAL OR
INTRATHECAL USE

Each mL contains morphine sulfate 15 mg, monobasic sodium phosphate, monohydrate 10 mg, dibasic sodium phosphate, anhydrous 2.8 mg, sodium formaldehyde sulfoxylate 3 mg and phenol 2.5 mg in Water for Injection. pH 2.5–6.5, sulfuric acid added, if needed, for pH adjustment. Sealed under nitrogen. USUAL DOSAGE: See package insert.

FOR INVENTORY ONLY — APPROXIMATION
15 mL 10 mL 5 mL

PROTECT FROM LIGHT
NOTE: Do not use if color is darker than pale yellow, if it is discolored in any other way or if it contains a precipitate. Store at 15°–30°C (59°–86°F). Avoid freezing. Caution: Federal law prohibits dispensing without prescription. Product Code: 2345-41
A-2345b
LOT   EXP.

ELKINS-SINN, INC. Cherry Hill, NJ 08003-4099
A subsidiary of A. H. Robins Company

a. Generic name _____

b. Dosage strength _____

c. Total quantity _____

d. Routes of administration _____

e. Controlled substance?   yes _____   no _____

f. Single dose vial?   yes _____   no _____

g. Ordered: Morphine sulfate 10 mg SC.
(Work problem to the thousandths place and round to the hundredths place).

The nurse will give_____

5.

60 mL   NDC 0003-0588-60
100,000 units per mL
MYCOSTATIN®
ORAL SUSPENSION
Nystatin Oral
Suspension USP
SHAKE WELL BEFORE USING
Caution: Federal law prohibits dispensing without prescription
☐APOTHECON®
A BRISTOL-MYERS SQUIBB COMPANY

Before Dispensing Replace Cap With Safety Cap Dropper.
Each mL contains 100,000 USP Nystatin Units in a vehicle containing 50% sucrose. Not more than 1% alcohol by volume. Usual dosage: See insert. Store at room temperature; avoid freezing.
APOTHECON®
A Bristol-Myers Squibb Company
Princeton, NJ 08540 USA   P1874-01

Ordered: Mycostatin susp. 1 million U p.o.
The nurse will give_____

6.

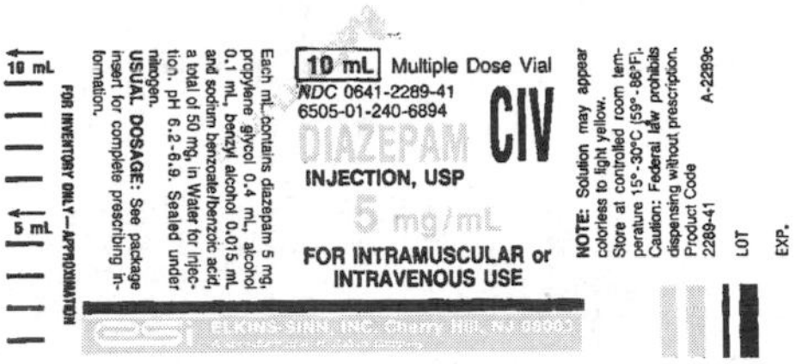

Label text (Diazepam vial):
10 mL Multiple Dose Vial
NDC 0641-2289-41
6505-01-240-6894
DIAZEPAM CIV
INJECTION, USP
5 mg/mL
FOR INTRAMUSCULAR or INTRAVENOUS USE
ELKINS-SINN, INC. Cherry Hill, NJ 08003

a. Generic name _____

b. Dosage strength _____

c. Routes of administration _____

d. Controlled substance?   yes _____   no _____

e. Single dose vial?   yes _____   no _____

f. Ordered: Diazepam 12.5 mg IM.

   The nurse will give_____

7.

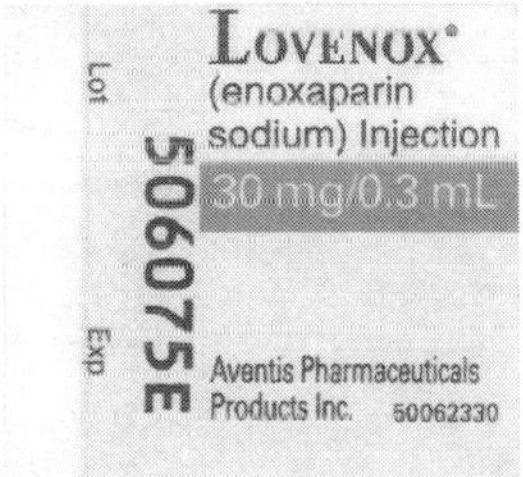

Label text (Lovenox):
LOVENOX®
(enoxaparin sodium) Injection
30 mg/0.3 mL
Lot 506075E
Aventis Pharmaceuticals Products Inc. 50062330

a. Trade name _____

b. Dosage strength _____

c. Route of administration _____

d. Storage information _____

8.

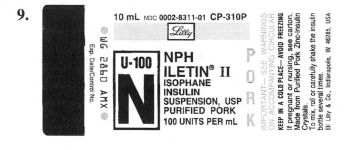

LOT

EXP.

To open—Cut seal along dotted line.

25 DOSETTE® Vials

Each contains **1 mL**

MEPERIDINE CII

HCl INJECTION, USP

75 mg/mL

WARNING: May be habit forming.

FOR INTRAMUSCULAR,
SUBCUTANEOUS OR
SLOW INTRAVENOUS USE

NDC 0641-**0150-25**

Each mL contains meperidine hydrochloride 75 mg, sodium metabisulfite
1.5 mg and phenol 5 mg in Water
for Injection. Buffered with acetic
acid-sodium acetate. pH 3.5-6.0.
Sealed under nitrogen.
USUAL DOSAGE: See package insert.
Do not use if precipitated.
Store at controlled room temperature 15°-30°C (59°-86°F).
Caution: Federal law prohibits dispensing without prescription.
Product Code: 0150-25   B-50150i

NDC3-0641-0150-25-1

ELKINS-SINN, INC. Cherry Hill, NJ 08003-4099
A subsidiary of A. H. Robins Company

a. Generic name _____

b. Dosage strength _____

c. Routes of administration _____

d. Controlled substance?   yes _____   no _____

e. Ordered: Meperidine 60 mg IM.

   The nurse will give_____

9.

10 mL NDC 0002-8311-01 CP-310P

Lilly

U-100

N

**NPH
ILETIN® II**
ISOPHANE
INSULIN
SUSPENSION, USP
PURIFIED PORK
100 UNITS PER mL

Exp. Date/Control No.   AMX 0860 GMG

IMPORTANT— SEE WARNINGS
ON ACCOMPANYING CIRCULAR
KEEP IN A COLD PLACE— AVOID FREEZING
If pregnant or nursing, see carton.
Made from Purified Pork Zinc-Insulin
Crystals.
To mix, roll or carefully shake the insulin
bottle several times.
Eli Lilly & Co., Indianapolis, IN 46285, USA

P O R K

a. Trade name _____

b. Insulin source _____

10.

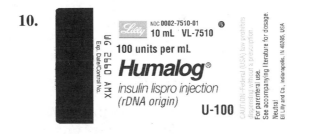

NDC 0002-7510-01 ®
10 mL VL-7510
100 units per mL
Humalog®
insulin lispro injection
(rDNA origin)
U-100

a. **Trade name** _____

b. **Ordered: Humalog 6 U SC now.**

The nurse will give_____

11.

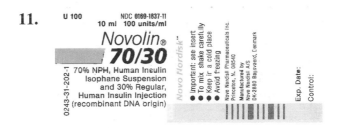

U 100   NDC 0169-1837-11
10 ml   100 units/ml
Novolin®
70/30
70% NPH, Human Insulin
Isophane Suspension
and 30% Regular,
Human Insulin Injection
(recombinant DNA origin)

a. **Trade name** _____

b. **Ordered: Novolin 70/30   22 U SC now.**

The nurse will give_____

12.

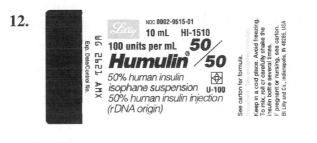

NDC 0002-9515-01
10 mL   HI-1510
100 units per mL **50/**
Humulin® **/50**
50% human insulin
isophane suspension U-100
50% human insulin injection
(rDNA origin)

Trade name _____

Module: ADMINISTRATION OF ORAL MEDICATIONS

ADMINISTRATION OF ORAL MEDICATIONS

KEY POINTS:

- In setting up oral medication problems, be sure that the units in the medication order and the available drug match.
- Use a conversion table to convert unlike units of measurement.
- When you arrive at the answer, ask yourself whether the answer is realistic. Nurses generally administer only 1–2 tablets and less than 30 cc of medication per dose.

<u>Working with Administration of Oral Medications</u>
Solve the following problems using the method of your choice.

1. The physician prescribed 0.8 mg of folic acid qd. The pharmacy sends 0.4 mg tablets. How many tablets will the nurse give?

    _____

2. The doctor orders acarbose 50 mg p.o. for the patient. How many tablets will the nurse give?

    _____

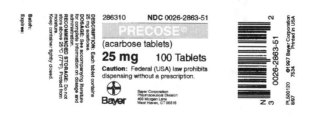

286310   NDC 0026-2863-51

PRECOSE®
(acarbose tablets)
25 mg   100 Tablets

Caution: Federal (USA) law prohibits dispensing without a prescription.

Bayer Corporation
Pharmaceutical Division
400 Morgan Lane
West Haven, CT 06516

DESCRIPTION: Each tablet contains 25 mg acarbose.
DOSAGE: See accompanying literature for complete information on dosage and administration.
RECOMMENDED STORAGE: Do not store above 25°C (77°F). Protect from moisture. Keep container tightly closed.

Batch:
Expires:

0026-2863-51

©1997 Bayer Corporation
Printed in USA
7534
PL500120
8/97

3. The order is for Zantac 0.15 g tabs i p.o. How many tablets will the nurse give to the patient?

_____

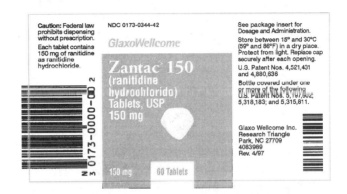

4. Lanoxin 0.125 mg is ordered stat. The pharmacy sends 0.25 mg tablets of Lanoxin. How many tablets will the nurse administer?

_____

5. Levothyroxine 0.1 mg is ordered q.o.d. The pharmacy sends 50 mcg tablets. How many tablets will the nurse give?

_____

6. Aluminum hydroxide suspension 15 cc is ordered q.i.d. Pharmacy sends a bottle of aluminum hydroxide labeled 320 mg/5 mL. How many mg is the patient receiving per dose?

_____

7. The patient receives furosemide 80 mg p.o. b.i.d.
   The pharmacy sends furosemide oral solution
   labeled 10 mg/mL. How many mL will the nurse
   give per dose?

   _____

8. The nurse is instructing a patient to take Paxil
   10 mg oral suspension at home. How many tsp will
   the nurse instruct the patient to take per dose?

   _____

Store at or below 25°C (77°F).
Keep tightly closed.
Shake well before using.
Each 5 mL contains paroxetine
hydrochloride equivalent to
10 mg paroxetine.
Dosage: See accompanying
prescribing information.
Caution: Federal law prohibits
dispensing without prescription.
Manufactured in Crawley, UK by
**SmithKline Beecham
Pharmaceuticals** for
**SmithKline Beecham
Pharmaceuticals**
Philadelphia, PA 19101

10mg/5mL
NDC 0029-3215-48

PAXIL®
PAROXETINE HCI
ORAL SUSPENSION

250 mL

LOT
EXP.

40163US1
40163US1
40163US1

670826-A

3 0029-3215-48 9

SB SmithKline Beecham

9. Diphenhydramine hydrochloride elixir 50 mg p.o.
   p.r.n. for itching is ordered. Diphenhydramine
   hydrochloride elixir 12.5 mg/5 mL is available.
   How many mL will the nurse give?

   _____

10. The order is for atropine gr 1/150 p.o. 1 hour
    before surgery. The pharmacy sends atropine
    0. 4-mg tablets. How many tablets will the nurse
    give?

    _____

11. The nurse practitioner orders nystatin 200,000 units p.o. q.i.d. p.c. swish and swallow. The pharmacy sends nystatin 100,000 units/5 mL. How many mL will the nurse give?

_____

12. Nitroglycerin p.o. gr 1/100 tablets is ordered p.r.n. for chest pain. Pharmacy sends nitroglycerin tablets labeled 0.3 mg/tablet. How many tablets will the nurse give?

_____

13. Cefaclor oral suspension 125 mL q.8h. is ordered for the patient upon discharge. The pharmacy sends the following bottle. How many days will this bottle last the patient?

_____

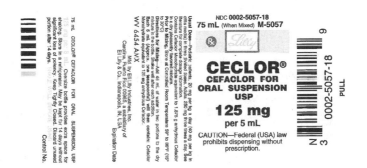

14. The doctor orders enalapril 0.0025 g p.o. q.d. Enalapril is available in 5 mg scored tablets. How many tablets will the nurse give?

_____

15. The order is for cyanocobalamin 1 mg p.o q.d. The pharmacy sends cyanocobalamin 1000 mcg tablets. How tablets will the nurse give?

_____

16. Aspirin gr xv p.o. is ordered p.r.n. for headache. Aspirin is available in 0.5 g scored tablets. How many tablets will the nurse administer?

_____

17. Codeine is available in 15 mg/5 mL. The order is for codeine 0.06 g   How many mL will the nurse give?

_____

18. The patient is to receive 20 mEq of KCl p.o. q.AM. The pharmacy sends a bottle labeled 30 mEq/15 mL. How many mL will the nurse administer?

_____

19. Morphine sulfate oral solution 120 mg q.4h. around the clock is ordered for a hospice patient. Morphine sulfate is available in 100 mg/5 mL. How many mg of morphine sulfate will the patient receive per day?

_____

20. Codeine gr s̄s̄ p.o. is ordered. Codeine is available in 30-mg tablets. How many tablets will the nurse give?

_____

Module: SYRINGES AND NEEDLES

SYRINGES

KEY POINTS:
- The most commonly used syringe, the 3-cc syringe, is calibrated to measure 0.1 cc accurately. Most 3 cc syringes have both minim and cc scales.
- The TB syringe measures volumes of 1 cc or less, and is calibrated to measure 0.01 cc accurately. The TB syringe has minim and cc scales.
- Larger volume syringes are calibrated in 0.2 or 1 cc increments.
- Insulin is measured in units and is drawn up in an insulin syringe. The standard insulin syringe is calibrated by 2 U increments. Low dosage insulin syringes are calibrated in 1 U increments.

Working with Syringes
Shade in the syringe with the amount of medication indicated.

1. **0.3 mL**

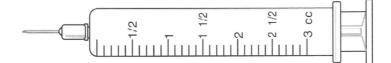

2. **0.66 mL**

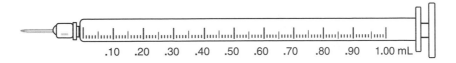

Copyright © 2002, F. A. Davis Company

3. 0.09 mL

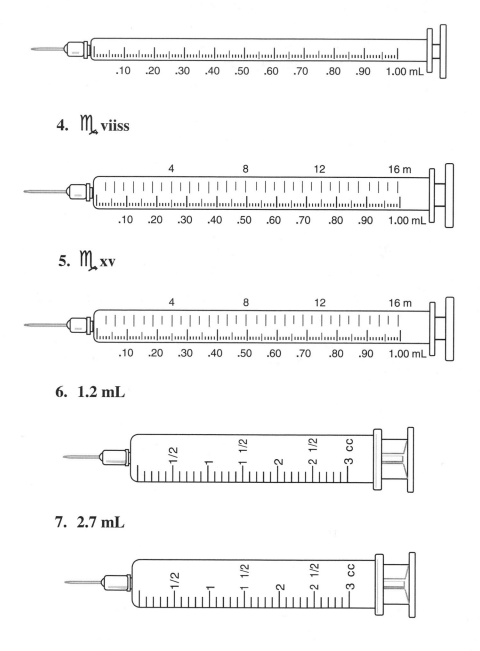

4. ℳ viiss

5. ℳ xv

6. 1.2 mL

7. 2.7 mL

8. 0.37 mL

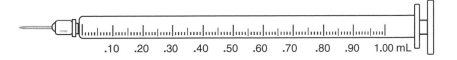

9. 1.9 mL

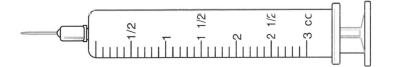

10. 4.6 mL

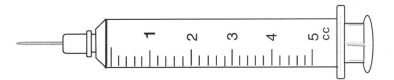

11. 38 units

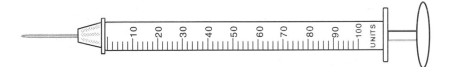

12. 27 units

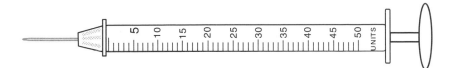

13. 7 units

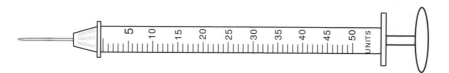

14. 7 units

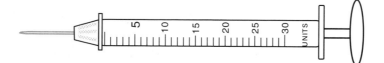

15. 16 units

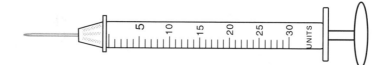

16. 56 units

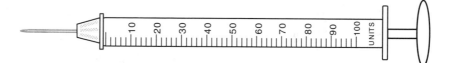

17. 3.8 mL

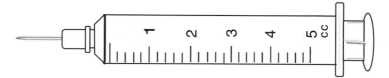

NEEDLES

KEY POINTS:
- Needles are identified by two numbers: length and gauge.
- Needle length is measured in inches.
- Needle gauge refers to the diameter. The larger the number of the gauge, the smaller the diameter of the needles.
- Needles are packaged in standard sizes with syringes for IM, ID, SC, and IV use.

<u>Working with Needles</u>
Choose the correct needle size for the following injections.

28 6 1/2"

1. A SC injection of insulin _____

2. An IM injection *21-33 1 1/2*

3. A TB skin test *26-27 3/8*

4. An IM injection to an obese person *21-23 2"*

5. A SC injection into the upper arm *25 5/8*

6. Drawing up viscous medication from a vial

_____

Choose the correct syringe and needle for the following injections. Fill in the syringe.

1. Meperidine 75 mg (1 mL) IM

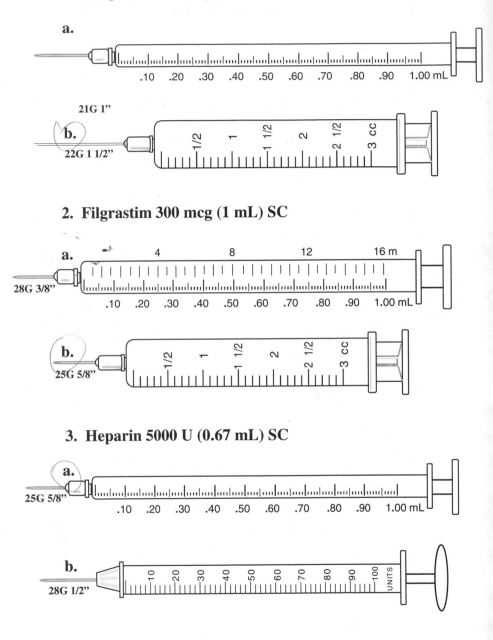

a.

.10   .20   .30   .40   .50   .60   .70   .80   .90   1.00 mL

21G 1"

b.

22G 1 1/2"

1/2   1   1 1/2   2   2 1/2   3 cc

2. Filgrastim 300 mcg (1 mL) SC

a.

4   8   12   16 m

28G 3/8"

.10   .20   .30   .40   .50   .60   .70   .80   .90   1.00 mL

b.

25G 5/8"

1/2   1   1 1/2   2   2 1/2   3 cc

3. Heparin 5000 U (0.67 mL) SC

a.

25G 5/8"

.10   .20   .30   .40   .50   .60   .70   .80   .90   1.00 mL

b.

28G 1/2"

10   20   30   40   50   60   70   80   90   100   UNITS

4. Hepatitis A vaccine 1 mL IM

a.

18G 1/2"

b.

23G 1 1/2"

5. Ketorolac 60 mg (2 mL) IM

a.

21G 1 1/2"   .10 .20 .30 .40 .50 .60 .70 .80 .90 1.00 mL

b.

22G 1 1/2"

6. Regular insulin 17 U SC

a.

28G 1/2"

b.

28G 1/2"

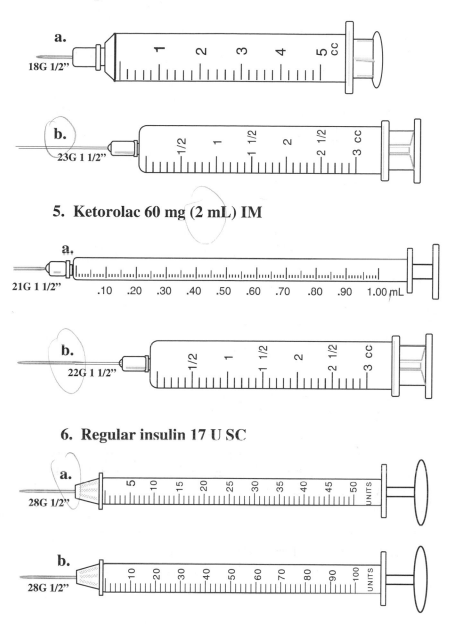

7. Regular insulin 6 U and NPH insulin 13 U SC

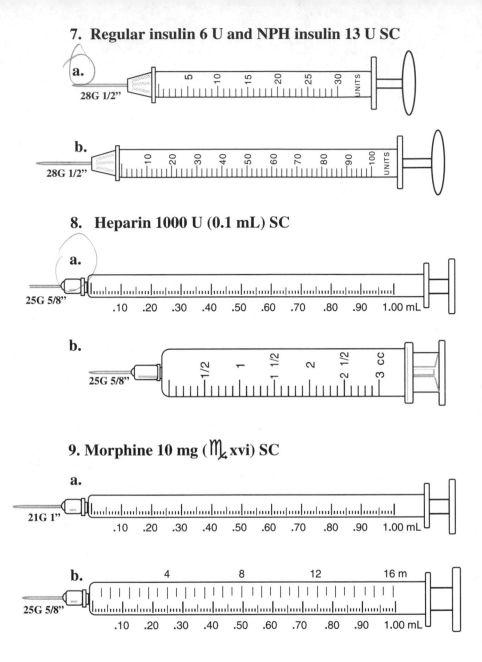

a.

28G 1/2"

5 10 15 20 25 30 UNITS

b.

28G 1/2"

10 20 30 40 50 60 70 80 90 100 UNITS

8. Heparin 1000 U (0.1 mL) SC

a.

25G 5/8"

.10 .20 .30 .40 .50 .60 .70 .80 .90 1.00 mL

b.

25G 5/8"

1/2 1 1 1/2 2 2 1/2 3 cc

9. Morphine 10 mg (℥ xvi) SC

a.

21G 1"

.10 .20 .30 .40 .50 .60 .70 .80 .90 1.00 mL

b.

25G 5/8"

4 8 12 16 m

.10 .20 .30 .40 .50 .60 .70 .80 .90 1.00 mL

Module: ADMINISTRATION OF PARENTERAL MEDICATIONS

ADMINISTRATION OF PARENTERAL MEDICATIONS

KEY POINTS:
- In setting up parenteral medication problems, be sure that the units in the medication order and the available drug match.
- Use a conversion table to convert unlike units of measurement.
- When you arrive at the answer, ask yourself whether the answer is realistic. Nurses generally administer 3 mL or less of a parenteral medication.
- With insulin, just draw up the total units ordered.

Working with Administration of Parenteral Medications
Use of method of your choice to solve the problems.

1. The physician prescribed 0.1 mg of folic acid IM. The pharmacy sends the following ampule. How many mL will the nurse give?

   _____

   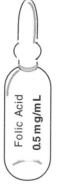

2. Meperidine HCl 75 mg is ordered stat. Meperidine HCl 50 mg/mL is available. How many mL will the nurse administer?

   _____

3. Heparin sodium 5000 U SC q.12h. is ordered for the patient. The pharmacy sends a vial labeled heparin sodium 20,000 U/mL. How many mL will the nurse give?

   _____

4. Procaine penicillin G 1.2 million U IM is ordered for the patient. The pharmacy sends procaine penicillin G 600,000 U/mL. How many mL will the nurse give?

   _____

   Fill in the syringe.

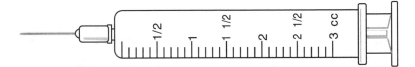

5. The preoperative order is meperidine HCl 60 mg with glycopyrrolate 0.08 mg IM stat. Meperidine HCl 100 mg/mL and glycopyrrolate 200 mcg/mL are available in the medication drawer. Calculate the preoperative medications.

   Meperidine HCl: _____

   Glycopyrrolate: _____

   Fill in the syringe with the total amount.

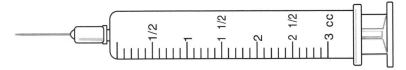

6. **Hydromorphone gr 1/60 SC q.3h. p.r.n. for pain is ordered for the patient. Hydromorphone 10 mg/mL is available in the narcotic drawer. How many mL will the nurse give?**

$$\frac{1}{60} \text{ gr } , \frac{60 \text{ mg}}{1 \text{ gr}} = 1 \text{ mg} \cdot \frac{1 \text{ mL}}{10 \text{ mg}} = 0.1 \text{ mL}$$

D

Fill in the ordered dose in each syringe.

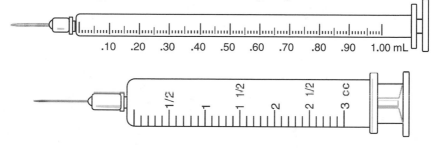

7. **The order is for atropine gr 1/150 SC now. The pharmacy sends the following vial. How many mL will the nurse give?**

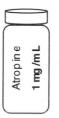

Atropine 1 mg/mL

_____

8. **The physician orders morphine sulfate 0.015 g. Morphine sulfate is available in 15 mg/mL. How many mimins will the nurse give?**

_____

Fill in the syringe.

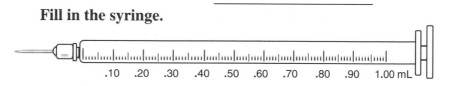

9. **Epoetin 12,000 U SC 3x/week is ordered. The pharmacy sends a vial of epoetin labeled 20,000 U/mL. How many mL will the nurse give?**

_____

Fill in the ordered dose in each syringe.

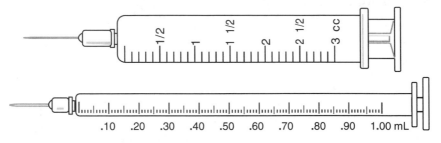

10. **The doctor orders ampicillin 250 mg. The pharmacy sends a vial of ampicillin labeled 1 g/mL. How many mL will the nurse give?**

_____

Fill in the ordered dose in the more appropriate syringe.

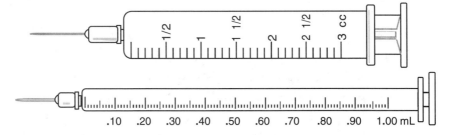

11. **The physician orders phenytoin 125 mg IM. The nurse prepares to draw up the medication from a vial labeled phenytoin 50 mg/mL. How many mL will the nurse give?**

_____

12. Humulin NPH insulin 23 U q.AM is ordered for the patient. How much insulin will the nurse give?

Fill in the more appropriate syringe.

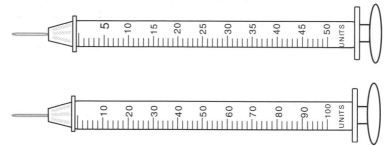

13. Humulin Lente insulin 35 U and Humulin Regular insulin 17 U q.AM is ordered for the patient. How much insulin will the nurse give?

Fill in the more appropriate syringe.

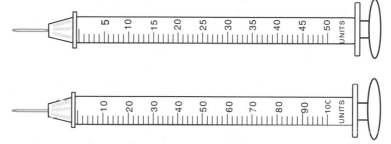

14. Humulin 70/30 insulin 21 U q.AM is ordered for the patient. How much insulin will the nurse give?

Fill in the more appropriate syringe.

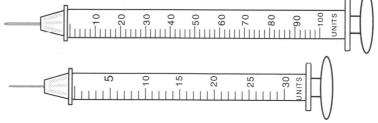

15. **Humulin 50/50 insulin 19 U q.AM is ordered for the patient. How much insulin will the nurse give?**

    Fill in the more appropriate syringe.

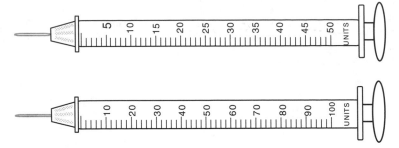

16. **Humulin Regular insulin 2 U is ordered for the patient. How much insulin will the nurse give?**

    Fill in the more appropriate syringe.

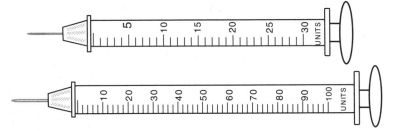

17. **Humulin NPH insulin 22 U and Humulin Regular insulin 7 U is ordered stat. How much insulin will the nurse give?**

    Fill in the more appropriate syringe.

Module: RECONSTITUTION OF POWDERED MEDICATIONS

SINGLE-STRENGTH RECONSTITUTION

KEY POINTS:

- In single-strength reconstitution, the manufacturer identifies one amount of diluent to add to the powdered medication.
- The dosage strength of the mixed medication is used to calculate the amount to give to the patient.
- Information needed to work with single-strength reconstitution problems includes the type and amount of diluent, the dosage strength of the mixed medication, the length of time the solution will remain stable, and storage information.
- Once the medication is reconstituted, the nurse writes the date and time of reconstitution and the nurse's initials on the medication label.

<u>Working with Single-Strength Reconstitution</u>
Solve the following single-strength reconstitution problems.

1. The physician orders cefazolin sodium 0.25 g IM q.8h. The pharmacy sends a 1 g vial of sterile cefazolin powder with the following mixing instructions: "For IM use, add 2.5 mL sterile water for injection and shake. Provides a volume of 3.0 mL (330 mg/mL)."

    a. How much diluent will be added to the cefazolin sodium powder?

    _____

b. What type of diluent will be added?

_____

c. What is the dosage strength of the mixed medication?

_____

d. How many mL of the medication will the nurse give to the patient?

_____

2. The order is for procaine penicillin G 300,000 units IM b.i.d. A 1-g vial of procaine penicillin G powder is in the medication drawer. The medication has the following mixing instructions: "IM use: Dissolve 4.6 mL bacteriostatic water for injection to make 200,000 units/mL."

a. How much diluent will be added to the procaine penicillin G powder?

_____

b. What type of diluent will be added?

_____

c. What is the dosage strength of the mixed medication?

_____

d. How many mL of the medication will the nurse give to the patient?

_____

3. **What data should be entered on the vial below when labeling the vial after reconstitution?**

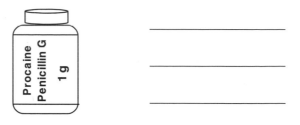

_____

_____

_____

4. **The physician orders 200 mg of an antibiotic IM q.12h. The pharmacy sends a vial of antibiotic powder for reconstitution with the following mixing directions: "For IM injection, IV direct (bolus) injection, or IV infusion, add 2 mL sterile water for injection. Shake well. Provides an approximate concentration of 125 mg/mL."**

a. **How much diluent will be added to the antibiotic powder?**

_____

b. **What type of diluent will be added?**

_____

c. **What is the dosage strength of the mixed medication?**

_____

d. **How many mL of the medication will the nurse give to the patient?**

_____

5. The order is for ticarcillin disodium 0.5 g IM q.6h. The directions state to add 2 mL of NS. The reconstituted solution contains 1 g/2.6 mL.

   a. What is the dosage strength of the reconstituted medication?

   1g / 2.6 ml

   b. How much will be given to the patient?

   0.5 g / 1.3 ml

6. The order is for oxacillin 450 mg IM q.6h.

NDC 0015-7981-20
EQUIVALENT TO
1 gram OXACILLIN
OXACILLIN SODIUM
FOR INJECTION, USP
Buffered—For IM or IV Use
CAUTION: Federal law prohibits
dispensing without prescription.
APOTHECON®
A BRISTOL-MYERS SQUIBB COMPANY

This vial contains oxacillin sodium monohydrate equivalent to 1 gram oxacillin and 20 mg dibasic sodium phosphate. Add 5.7 mL Sterile Water for Injection, USP • Each 1.5 mL contains 250 mg oxacillin. • Usual Dosage: Adults—250 mg to 500 mg Intramuscularly every 4 to 6 hours. See circular for intravenous use. READ ACCOMPANYING CIRCULAR Discard solution after 3 days at room temperature or 7 days under refrigeration.
APOTHECON®
A Bristol-Myers Squibb Company
Princeton, NJ 08540 USA

798120DRL-2

Cont:
Exp. Date:

   a. How much diluent will be added to the oxacillin powder?

   5.7 ml

   b. What type of diluent will be added?

   SW

   c. What is the resulting dosage strength of the mixed medication?

   1.5 ml 250 mg

   d. How many mL of the oxacillin will the nurse give to the patient?

   2.7 ml

7. The physician orders Augmentin 500 mg p.o. q.12h. The pharmacy sends the following drug:

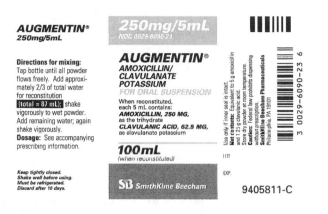

a. How much diluent will be added to the Augmentin powder?

_____

b. What is the dosage strength of the mixed medication?

_____

c. How many mL of the Augmentin oral suspension will the nurse give to the patient?

_____

d. What data should be entered on the label above after reconstitution?

_____

_____

_____

MULTIPLE-STRENGTH RECONSTITUTION

KEY POINTS:
- **In multiple-strength reconstitution, the manufacturer identifies several amounts of diluent to add to the powdered medication.**
- **The nurse must select one of the listed amounts of diluent.**
- **The dosage strength of the mixed medication is used to calculate the amount to give to the patient.**
- **Information needed to work with multiple-strength reconstitution problems includes the type and amount of diluent, the dosage strength of the mixed medication, the length of time the solution will remain stable, and storage information.**
- **Once the medication is reconstituted, the nurse circles the amount of diluent selected and the corresponding dosage strength. The date and time of reconstitution and the nurse's initials are also written on the medication label.**

Working with Multiple-Strength Reconstitution
Solve the following multiple-strength reconstitution problems.

1. When preparing multiple-strength reconstitution medications, the nurse will make the most concentrated solution when adding:

   ☐ the largest volume of diluent.

   ☐ the smallest volume of diluent.

2. The physician orders cefoperazone 750 mg IV q.12h. The pharmacy sends a 2 g vial of sterile cefoperazone powder with the following mixing instructions: "Diluent: sterile bacteriostatic water for injection. Add 10 mL for an approximate volume of 100 mg/mL. Add 15 mL for an approximate volume of 150 mg/mL.

a. What is the dosage strength if the nurse chooses to add 10 mL of diluent?

_____

b. How many mL of the mixed solution will the nurse administer to the patient?

_____

c. What information needs to be written on the label of the reconstituted cefoperazone?

_____
_____
_____
_____

3. The physician orders penicillin G potassium 1 million U IV q.6h. The nurse has a vial with the following instructions:

Add Diluent (mL)	Dosage Strength of Mixed Medication
9.6	100,000 U/mL
4.6	200,000 U/mL
1.6	500,000 U/mL

a. What is the dosage strength if the nurse chooses to add 9.6 mL of diluent?

_____

b. What is the dosage strength if the nurse chooses to add 1.6 mL of diluent?

_____

c. Select one volume of diluent, and calculate the amount of penicillin G potassium to administer.

_____

4. The physician orders 750,000 U of penicillin G potassium. The nurse has the following vial:

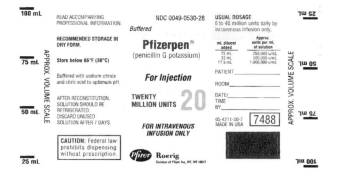

a. Select one volume of diluent. What is the dosage strength of the mixed medication if this volume of diluent is added to the vial?

_____

b. Calculate the amount of medication to administer.

_____

c. How long is the solution stable if refrigerated?

_____

d. Complete the label with the correct information.

5. The physician orders ampicillin 700 mg IV q.6h. The nurse has a vial of powdered ampicillin with the following directions for reconstitution:

For IM or IV use: Add bacteriostatic NS or sterile water for injection and shake.

Diluent	Strength of Mixed Medication
3.5 mL	500 mg/mL
7.2 mL	250 mg/mL

Use within 1 hour of reconstitution. Stable under refrigeration for 6 hours. See package insert.

a. Select one volume of diluent. What is the dosage strength of the mixed medication if this volume of diluent is added to the vial?

_____

b. Calculate the amount of medication to administer.   _____

c. How long is the mixed solution stable?

_____

d. If the ampicillin is given IM, which diluent volume would be preferable? Why?

_____

e. Complete the label with the appropriate information.

Module: IV CALCULATIONS

Working with Milliliters per Hour

Solve the following problems using the method of your choice.

1. The order is for 1000 cc D5/0.225 NS q.12h. How many cc/hr will the nurse set on the IV pump?

_____

2. The order is for 1000 cc D5/W q.16h. How many cc/hr will the nurse set on the IV pump?

_____

3. The physician orders 3000 cc Ringer's lactate to infuse over 24 hours. How many mL will the patient receive per hour?

_____

4. The order is to infuse 1 U of packed red blood cells (250 cc) over 1 1/2 hours. Calculate the mL/hr.

_____

5. The doctor orders ceftizoxime 1 g IVPB q.12h. The pharmacy sends ceftizoxime 1 g in 50 cc NS to infuse over 30 minutes. Calculate the mL/hr.

_____

6. The physician orders 1 L 0.9% NS to infuse over 6 hours. Calculate the mL/hr.

_____

7. The order is to infuse 500 cc of D5W over 10 hrs. Calculate the many mL/hr.

_____

Working with Flow Rate

1. The nurse hangs up 1 L D5W to infuse over 8 hours. Use the following IV tubing label to calculate the flow rate.

_____

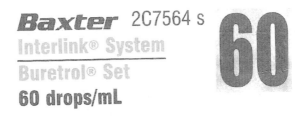

Baxter 2C7564 s
Interlink® System
Buretrol® Set
60 drops/mL

2. The physician orders 1 L of D5LR to infuse at 83 cc/hr. The IV tubing delivers 15 gtt/cc. What is the flow rate (gtt/min)?

   _____

3. The doctor orders 1 U of whole blood (500 cc) to infuse over 4 hours. The blood tubing delivers 10 gtt/cc. What is the flow rate of the blood?

   _____

4. The order is for 500 mL of NS TKO (30 mL/hr). The nurse selects the following IV tubing. What is the flow rate?

   _____

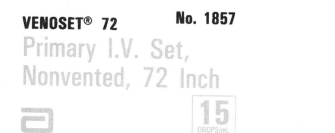

VENOSET® 72   **No. 1857**

Primary I.V. Set,
Nonvented, 72 Inch

15 DROPS/mL

5. The IV is to infuse at 42 cc/hr. The drop factor on the IV tubing is 15 gtt/mL. What is the flow rate?

   _____

6. The order is to infuse 250 cc of NS over 1 1/2 hours. The drop factor is 12 gtt/mL. What is the flow rate?

   _____

IV PUSH MEDICATIONS

KEY POINTS:
- Use a drug reference book to find the rate of administration for IV push medications.
- If the dosage ordered is smaller than the recommended dose in the drug reference book, administer the dosage over the full amount of time recommended.
- The term "fraction thereof" in a drug reference book means that any fraction of a dose is given over the full amount of time recommended.

Working with IV Push Medication
Use the information provided to identify the IV push rate of administration for the following problems.

1. The doctor orders morphine sulfate 10 mg IVP stat. The recommended rate of administration is 15 mg or fraction thereof over 4–5 minutes. What is the rate of administration for this dose?

   _____

2. The doctor orders hydromorphone 3 mg IV for severe pain. The drug reference literature states "Administer slowly at a rate not to exceed 2 mg over 3–5 min. Rapid infusion may lead to respiratory depression, hypotension, and circulatory collapse." What is the rate of administration for this dose?

   _____

3. The doctor orders furosemide 80 mg IVP now. What is the rate of administration for this dose?

_____

DIURETICS (LOOP)

furosemide
(fur-**oh**-se-mide)

IMPLEMENTATION

- **Direct IV: Administer undiluted.**
  Rate: Administer slowly over 1–2 minutes.
- **Intermittent Infusion: Dilute large doses . . .**
  Rate: Not to exceed 4 mg/min.

---

4. The doctor orders methylprednisolone sodium succinate 250 mg IVP q.d. The recommended rate of administration is 500 mg over 2–3 minutes or longer. What is the rate of administration for this dose?

_____

5. The doctor orders diazepam 10 mg IVP now. The drug book states "Administer slowly at a rate of 5 mg over at least 1 minute." What is the rate of administration for this dose?

_____

6. The doctor orders lorazepam 0.001 g IVP 30 minutes before chemotherapy. What is the rate of administration for this dose?

_____

LORAZEPAM
(lor-**az**-e-pam)

IMPEMENTATION

- *Rate:* **Administer direct IV, through Y-site at a rate of 2 mg over 1 minute. Rapid IV administration may result in apnea, hypotension, bradycardia, or cardiac arrest.**

---

7. The doctor orders phenytoin 75 mg IVP for the patient experiencing status epilepticus. What is the rate of administration for this dose?

_____

PHENYTOIN
(**fen**-i-toyn)

IMPEMENTATION

Direct IV: Administer at a rate not to exceed 50 mg over 1 minute (25 mg/min [may be as low as 5–10 mg/min] in patients who may develop hypotension . . .).

INFUSION AND COMPLETION TIME

KEY POINTS:
- Use cc/hr and total amount of IV fluid to calculate the infusion time (hours and minutes).
- Use the starting time and the infusion time to calculate the completion time of the IV fluid.
- With infusion time, convert parts of an hour to minutes.

Working with Infusion Time
Use the information provided to identify the infusion time for the following problems.

1. The doctor orders 1 L of D5/0.45 NS to infuse at 125 cc/hr. What is the infusion time of the IV?

   _____

2. At 0700, 500 cc of D5W is started to infuse at 60 cc/hr. What is the infusion time of the IV?

   _____

3. At 1000, 1000 cc of lactated Ringer's (LR) is started in the patient. The IV is infusing at 75 mL/hr. The drop factor is 10 gtt/min. What is the infusion time of the IV?

   _____

4. The nurse restarts an IV with 800 mL D5/LR to infuse at 125 cc/hr. What is the infusion time of the IV?

   _____

5. The patient has an IVPB of famotidine 20 mg in 100 mL NS. The nurse sets the IV pump at 200 mL/hr. What is the infusion time of the IVPB?

_____

6. The nurse starts an IV of 100 cc D5W with 10 mEq KCl to infuse at 30 cc/hr. What is the infusion time of the IV?

_____

Working with Completion Time

1. The nurse starts 1 L of D5/0.45 NS to infuse at 125 cc/hr at 0800. What is the completion time of this IV?

_____

2. At 1400, 250 cc of D5W is started to infuse at 60 cc/hr. What is the completion time of the IV?

_____

3. At 2000, 1000 cc of 0.45 NS is started to infuse at 100 mL/hr. What is the completion time of the IV?

_____

4. The nurse restarts an IV bag containing 600 cc of IV fluid at 1930 to infuse at 75 mL/hr. What is the completion time of the IV?

_____

5. The nurse restarts an IV bag containing 500 cc of D5/0.45 NS at 1430 to infuse at 80 cc/hr. What is the completion time of this IV?

_____

6. The nurse restarts 750 cc of LR at 0900 to infuse at 150 cc/hr. What is the completion time of the IV?

_____

Working with Infusion and Completion Time

1. The doctor orders 1 L NS to infuse over 10 hours. The nurse starts the IV at 0900. At 1000 the patient pulls out the IV. The nurse restarts the IV at 1100 at the same rate. Starting with the amount of IV fluid left at 1100, calculate the new infusion time and the completion time of the IV.

Infusion time_____

Completion time_____

2. The doctor orders 500 cc D10W to infuse at 75 cc/hr. The nurse starts the IV at 1330. At 1530 the IV rate is increased to 100 cc/hr per doctor's orders. Starting with the amount of IV fluid remaining at 1530, calculate the new infusion time and the completion time of the IV.

Infusion time_____

Completion time_____

3. The doctor orders 1 L NS to infuse over 8 hours. The nurse starts the IV at 1600. At 2000 the IV rate is decreased to 100 cc/hr. Starting with the amount of IV fluid remaining at 2000, calculate the new infusion time and the completion time of the IV.

Infusion time_____

Completion time_____

4. The doctor order 500 cc of NS to infuse at 100 cc/hr. The nurse starts the IV at 0530. At 0700 the IV rate is decreased to 75 cc/hr. Starting with the amount of IV fluid remaining at 0700, calculate the new infusion time and the completion time of the IV.

Infusion time_____

Completion time_____

5. At 1600, 1 L D5W is started to infuse over 8 hours. At 1900, the IV infiltrates. The nurse restarts the IV at 2100 at the same IV rate. Starting with the amount of IV fluid remaining at 2100, calculate the new infusion time and the completion time of the IV.

Infusion time_____

Completion time_____

```
┌─────────────────────────────────────────────┐
│┌───────────────────────────────────────────┐│
││              LABELING IV BAGS              ││
││                                            ││
││ KEY POINTS:                                ││
││ • When labeling a flowmeter, be sure to    ││
││   include the start time and end time of   ││
││   the IV.                                   ││
││ • Use military time to identify the hourly ││
││   fluid intake on the flowmeter.           ││
│└───────────────────────────────────────────┘│
└─────────────────────────────────────────────┘
```

LABELING IV BAGS

KEY POINTS:
- When labeling a flowmeter, be sure to include the start time and end time of the IV.
- Use military time to identify the hourly fluid intake on the flowmeter.

Labeling IV Bags
Label the following flowmeters to identify the IV fluid intake.

1. The doctor orders 1 L NS to infuse over 10 hours. The nurse starts the IV at 1100. Label the flowmeter with the hourly fluid intake.

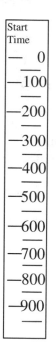

2. **The nurse starts the IV at 0230 to infuse at 75 cc/hr. Label the flowmeter hourly.**

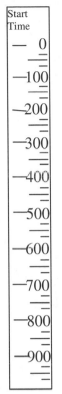

3. **The nurse starts the IV at 0100 at 50 cc/hr. Label the flowmeter q.2h.**

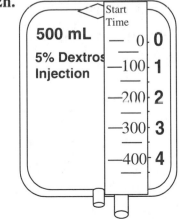

4. **The nurse starts the IV at 1300 to infuse at 150 cc/hr. Label the flowmeter hourly.**

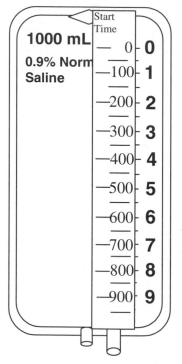

Shade in the amount of IV fluid in the bag at 1700.

5. **The nurse starts the IV at 2030 to infuse at 125 cc/hr. Label the flowmeter hourly.**

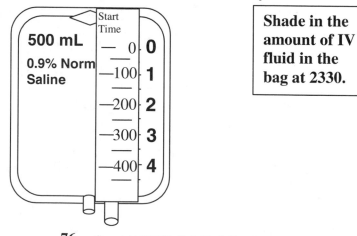

Shade in the amount of IV fluid in the bag at 2330.

Module: PEDIATRIC CALCULATIONS

ADMINISTERING MEDICATIONS TO CHILDREN

KEY POINTS:
- The oral route is preferred for children. Children over 5 years can take chewable forms of medication. Special equipment is available for oral pediatric administration.
- Parenteral doses for children are generally not rounded, but are left at the tenth or the hundredth place.
- The maximum volume of a parenteral injection in children is generally 1 mL. For the SC route, 0.5 mL is the maximum volume, and for the ID route, 0.01–0.1 mL is the maximum volume of the injection.
- Shorter length (1/2"–1") and smaller diameter (25G–30G) needles are used.
- The smallest possible amount of diluent is added to dilute pediatric IV medications. A pedidrip tubing (60 gtt/mL) and a burette may be used to administer pediatric IV fluids and medications.

Administering Medications to Children
Solve the following problems using the method of your choice.

1. The physician prescribed divalproex sodium 0.25 g q.d. p.o. Divalproex sodium is available from the pharmacy in 125 mg delayed-release tablets. How many tablets will the nurse give?

2. The child is to receive cefaclor 350 mg p.o. q.12h. The pharmacy sends strawberry-flavored cefaclor oral suspension in 125 mg/5mL strength. How many mL will the child receive per dose?

_____

3. The doctor orders phenobarbital 45 mg q.h.s. The nurse finds the following in the medication drawer. How many tablets will the nurse give?

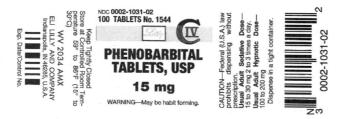

_____

4. The order is for 0.25 g of amoxicillin p.o. q.8h. for a 6-year-old child. The following medication is available. How many tablets will the nurse give?

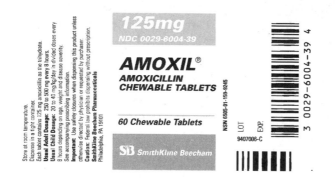

_____

5.a. Prochlorperazine 2.5 mg p.o. b.i.d. is ordered. The pharmacy sends prochlorperazine syrup 5 mg/5 mL. How much will the patient receive?

_____

b. Fill in the more appropriate measuring device for this medication.

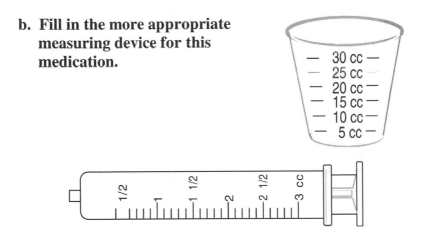

6.a. Methylprednisolone 20 mg IV q.12h. is ordered. The pharmacy sends the following medication. How many mL will the nurse administer per dose?

Single-Dose Vial
For intramuscular or intravenous use. See package insert for complete product information. Contains Benzyl Alcohol as a Preservative. Store solution at controlled room temperature 20° to 25° C (68° to 77° F) [see USP] and use within 48 hours after mixing. Protect from light.
Each 4 mL (when mixed) contains:
• Methylprednisolone sodium succinate equivalent to 500 mg methylprednisolone (125 mg per mL). Lyophilized in container.   813 974 305
Pharmacia & Upjohn Co., Kalamazoo, MI 49001, USA

NDC 0009-0765-02   4 mL Act-O-Vial®

Solu-Medrol®
methylprednisolone sodium succinate for injection, USP

500 mg*

_____

b. Fill in the syringe.

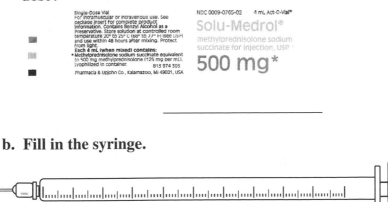

7.a. The physician orders IV tobramycin 12 mg q.12h. The pharmacy sends the following vial of tobramycin. How many mL will the nurse give?

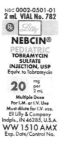

NDC 0002-0501-01
2 mL VIAL No. 782

Lilly

NEBCIN®
PEDIATRIC
TOBRAMYCIN
SULFATE
INJECTION, USP
Equiv. to Tobramycin

20 mg
per
2 mL

Multiple Dose
For I.M. or I.V. Use
Must dilute for I.V. use.
Eli Lilly & Company
Indpls., IN 46285, U.S.A.
WW 1510 AMX
Exp. Date/Control No.

_____

b. The nurse dilutes the tobramycin in a burette with 30 mL D5W. The IV medication is to infuse over 30 minutes. How many mL/hr will the nurse set on the IV pump?

_____

8.a. The patient has a primary IV of D5/0.225 NS infusing by gravity flow at 75 mL/hr. The IV tubing is a pedidrip tubing. The physician orders ampicillin 250 mg in 50 mL D5W IV q.6h. The IVPB is to infuse over ½ hour. What is the flow rate of the IVPB?

_____

b. What time will the IVPB be completed if the nurse starts the IVPB at 1400?

_____

DETERMINING SAFE DOSE

KEY POINTS:

- In order to determine whether an ordered dose is safe for an individual child, the nurse needs the following information: the medication order, the child's weight (usually in kg) or body surface area (BSA), and the recommended dose from the drug reference book.

- Recommended drug dosages can be stated as individual doses (for example, mg/kg or mcg/m^2), total daily doses, or as dosage ranges. The nurse needs to read the drug reference book carefully to interpret the drug information correctly.

- After calculating the recommended dose based on a child's weight or BSA, it is compared with the ordered dose. An ordered dose is considered safe when it is equal to or smaller than the dose recommended in the drug reference book.

Dosage Based on Body Weight

Solve the following problems using the method of your choice.

1.a. The physician orders cefdinir 200 mg p.o. q.12h. for a child who weighs 30 kg. The drug reference book states that the recommended dose for children from 6 months to 12 years is 7 mg/kg q.12h. What is the maximum safe dose based on the drug literature for this child?

_____

b. Is the ordered dose safe?

_____

2.a. The physician orders a digitalizing dose of IV digoxin 0.25 mg p.o. q.12h. for a 12-month-old child who weighs 8 kg. The drug reference book states that the recommended digitalizing dose for children from 1–24 months is 30–50 mcg/kg. What is the maximum safe dose based on the drug literature for this child?

_____

b. Is the ordered dose safe?

_____

3.a. The physician orders furosemide oral solution 40 mg p.o. q.d. for a child who weighs 66 lb. The drug reference book states that the recommended dose of p.o. furosemide for children is 1–2 mg/kg as a single dose initially, up to 5–6 mg/kg/day. What is the maximum safe dose based on the drug literature for this child?

_____

b. Is the ordered dose safe?

_____

4.a. A child who weighs 77 lb is started on oral morphine solution 20 mg p.o. q.3h. The recommended dose of oral morphine for children < 50 kg is 0.3 mg/kg q.3–4h. initially. What is the maximum safe dose based on the drug literature for this child?

_____

b. Is the ordered dose safe?

_____

5.a. The order is for phenytoin sodium 125 mg IV
q.8h. for a 15-year-old patient with frequent
seizures. The patient weighs 55 kg. The drug
reference book states that the recommended
pediatric maintenance dose of phenytoin sodium
is 4–8 mg/kg/24 hr in divided doses every 8–12
hours. What is the maximum safe dose based
on the drug literature for this child?

_____

b. Is the ordered dose safe?

_____

Dosage Based on Body Surface Area
Solve the following problems using the method of your
choice.

1.a. A child who has a BSA of 0.8 m^2 is given
leucovorin calcium 5 mg q.6h. The drug reference
book states that the recommended dose for
children is 7 mg/ m^2 q.6h. What is the maximum
safe dose based on the drug literature for this
child?

_____

b. Is the ordered dose safe?

_____

2.a. An order is written for zidovudine 0.25 g p.o. q.6h. for a child who has a BSA of 1.1 m^2. The drug reference book states that the recommended dose for children from 3 months to 12 years is 90–180 mg/m^2 q.6h. What is the maximum safe dose based on the drug literature for this child?

_____

b. Is the ordered dose safe?

_____

3.a. The physician prescribes vinblastine 10 mg IV q.week for a child who weighs 75 lb and has a body surface area of 1.15 m^2. The drug reference book states that the recommended dose of vinblastine for children is 2.5 mg/m^2 as a single dose initially, up to 7.5 mg/m^2/q.1–2 weeks up to 12 weeks. What is the maximum safe based on the drug literature for this child?

_____

b. Is the ordered dose safe?

_____

4.a. The order is for 0.2 mg q.d. of a drug for a child with a BSA of 0.4 m^2. The recommended dose of the drug is 0.55 mg/m^2 q.d. What is the maximum safe dose based on the drug literature for this child?

_____

b. Is the ordered dose safe?

_____

5.a. An 11-year-old child with leukemia and an acute varicella zoster infection is started on acyclovir 500 mg IV q.8h. The child's BSA is 1.18 m^2. The recommended dose of acyclovir for immunosuppressed children < 12 years old with varicella zoster is 500 mg/m^2 q.8h. for 7 days.

_____

b. Is the ordered dose safe?

_____

Nasogastric Fluid Replacement

NASOGASTRIC FLUID REPLACEMENT

KEY POINTS:
- To calculate fluid replacement for a child with a large volume of NG drainage, the nurse needs the following information: the rate of the primary IV, the maximum hourly IV rate, the amount of NG drainage, and the time interval for measuring and replacing the output.
- NG fluid replacement problems usually involve solving for the infusion and completion time of the replacement IV fluid.

Working with Nasogastric Fluid Replacement Problems
Solve the following problems using the method of your choice.

1.a. A child with a NG tube to low continuous suction has an order for 1 L D5/0.225 NS @ 100 cc/hr. The NG drainage is to be measured q.8h. and replaced with a second IV of D5W with 10 mEq KCl per 500 cc. The child is to receive no more than 150 cc/hr IV. What is the rate of the primary IV?

_____

b. What is the maximum hourly IV rate?

_____

c. The child's NG tube drains 380 cc. What is the infusion time of the replacement IV?

_____

d. What is the completion time of the replacement IV if replacement is started at 1500?

_____

2.a. The order is for 500 mL D5/0.225 NS @ 63 mL/hr. The NG drainage is to be measured and replaced with the primary IV solution q.4h. Maximum hourly IV rate is not to exceed 85 mL/hr. What is the rate of the primary IV?

_____

b. The nurse can increase the IV how many additional mL/hr during the replacement of the NG drainage?

_____

c. The child's NG tube drains 66 cc. What is the infusion time of the replacement IV fluid?

_____

d. The fluid replacement is started at 12 noon. What is the completion time?

_____

3.a. The physician writes the following orders:
1. IV 500 mL 0.33 NS @ 75 cc/hr.
2. Replace NG drainage cc for cc q.4h. with 2nd IV of 0.45 NS with 10 mEq KCl per 500 cc. Maximum hourly IV rate—100 mL/hr.
The NG output at 0400 is 100 cc. What is the infusion time of the replacement IV?

_____

b. What is the completion time if the replacement IV is started at 0430?

_____

4.a. The physician writes the following orders:
1. IV 500 mL D5/0.225 NS q.10h.
2. Replace NG drainage cc for cc with the maintenance IV fluid q.4h.
3. Maximum hourly IV rate—80 mL/hr.
The NG output at 2200 is 135 mL. What is the infusion time of the replacement IV fluid?

_____

b. What is the completion time if the replacement IV is started at 2245?

_____

Module: TITRATION OF IV MEDICATIONS

TITRATION OF IV MEDICATIONS

KEY POINTS:
- With titration problems, the nurse usually needs to calculate the number of mL/hr to set on the IV pump. Occasionally the nurse needs to calculate the amount of medication infusing per hour.
- Information needed to solve titration problems includes the total drug, the total volume of IV fluid, and the amount of drug ordered to infuse hourly.
- Titration orders can be written as a dosage range or as a single dose of medication.

Solving Titration Problems
Solve the following titration problems.

1. Ordered: IV dobutamine 100 mcg/min
   Available: dobutamine 250 mg in 250 mL D5W
   The nurse is told in morning report that the patient is receiving 5 mL/hr via IV pump.

   a. Calculate the mg/hr.

   _____

   b. Calculate the mL/hr.

   _____

   c. Is the set dose correct?

   _____

2. Ordered: 1 mg lidocaine/min IV
   Available: 2 g lidocaine in 500 mL D5W

   a. Calculate the mg/hr.

   _____

b. Calculate the mL/hr.

   _____

c. If the lidocaine is increased to 2 mg/min, calculate the mL/hr.

   _____

3. Ordered: IV lidocaine 4 mg/min
   Available: 1 g lidocaine in 500 mL D5W

   a. Calculate the mL/hr.

      _____

   b. If the rate is reduced to 2 mg/min, calculate the mL/hr.

      _____

4. The pharmacy sends an IV of 125 mg diltiazem HCl in 500 mL D5W. The physician has ordered diltiazem HCl 5 mg/hr. Calculate the mL/hr.

   _____

5. Heparin 25,000 U in 250 cc D5W is sent up from the pharmacy. The order is to administer heparin at 1000 U/hr. How many mL/hr will the nurse set on the IV pump?

   _____

6. The pharmacy sends an IV of magnesium sulfate 22 g in 500 mL D5W. The order is for 50 mg/min. Calculate the mL/hr.

   _____

7. A patient with ventricular ectopic beats has stat orders for a lidocaine infusion at a rate of 30 mL/hr. The IV contains 1 g lidocaine in 500 mL D5W. Calculate the mg/hr that the patient will receive.

_____

8. One g of aminophylline is added to 500 mL NS. The order is to infuse the IV over 10 hours. Calculate the mg/hr that the patient will receive.

_____

9. Pronestyl 1 g in 250 mL NS is ordered for a patient with frequent PVCs to run at 1 mL/min. Calculate the mg/min that the patient is receiving.

_____

10. The doctor writes an order for heparin 1400 U/hr. The pharmacy sends an IV of 500 mL D5W with 20,000 units of heparin. What rate will the nurse set on the IV pump?

_____

11. The order is for IV dopamine HCl 400 mg in 500 mL NS. The patient is to receive 750 mcg/min. What rate will the nurse set on the IV pump?

_____

12. Ordered: Nitroglycerine 10 mcg/min IV
Available: Nitroglycerine 50 mg in 250 mL NS
What rate will the nurse set on the IV pump?

_____

13. The order is for IV dopamine HCl 400 mg/500 mL NS. The patient is to receive 500–750 mcg/min. What rate will the nurse set on the IV pump to administer the lowest dosage of dopamine HCl?

                            _____

14. The order is for IV NTG 5–100 mcg/min to relieve chest pain. NTG 50 mg in 250 mL NS is available. What rate will the nurse set on the IV pump to deliver the highest dosage?

                            _____

15. The physician orders dopamine 20 mcg/kg/min for a patient who weighs 80 kg. The pharmacy sends an IV of 400 mg of dopamine in 500 mL D5W. What rate will the nurse set on the IV pump?

                            _____

16. The physician orders milrinone lactate 0.5–0.75 mcg/kg/min IV for a patient with CHF who weighs 121 lb. The pharmacy sends an IV of 20 mg of milrinone lactate in 150 mL D5W. What rate will the nurse set on the IV pump to administer the lowest dosage?

                            _____

17. The physician orders IV morphine sulfate 2–5 mg/hr for pain management. The pharmacy sends an IV of 250 mg of morphine sulfate in 500 mL D5W. What rate will the nurse set on the IV pump to administer 3 mg/hr?

                            _____

18. The physician orders propranolol 1 mg/hr. The pharmacy sends an IV of 15 mg propranolol in 500 mL NS. Calculate the mL/hr.

_____

19.a. A patient with severe asthma who weighs 55 kg is started on an IV theophylline drip in the emergency room. An IV of 250 mg theophylline ethylenediamine in 500 mL NS is started at 1300. The order is to start the IV infusion at 0.5 mg/kg/hr. The dose to be increased as needed by 0.1 mg/kg/hr q.30 min up to a maximum of 0.7 mg/kg/hr. Calculate the mL/hr that the nurse will set on the infusion pump at 1300.

_____

b. If the theophylline drip is increased as ordered at 1330, what rate will be set on the IV pump?

_____

20.a. The patient has a dopamine drip running at 45 mL/hr. The order is for 400 mg dopamine HCl in 500 mL D5W to run at 5–15 mcg/kg/min. The nurse started the dopamine at 8 mcg/kg/min. The patient weighs 165 pounds. Is the correct rate set on the IV pump?

_____

b. If the rate is increased to 9 mcg/kg/min, what rate should be set on the IV pump?

_____

ANSWERS

Module: BASIC MATH REVIEW

Working with Addition of Fractions

1.	3/5	6.	15 5/24
2.	11/21	7.	14 4/45
3.	1 1/15	8.	15 1/10
4.	5 1/4	9.	17 5/8
5.	5 9/20	10.	21 3/4

Working with Subtraction of Fractions

1.	1/2	6.	2 1/2
2.	3/10	7.	4 21/40
3.	5/24	8.	10 11/24
4.	2 7/8	9.	10 19/42
5.	7 3/10	10.	7 1/10

Working with Multiplication of Fractions

1.	3/10	6.	14 16/21
2.	5/9	7.	3 3/16
3.	1/2	8.	11 11/35
4.	15/16	9.	22 11/24
5.	19 4/5	10.	3 13/54

Working with Division of Fractions

1.	1 2/5	6.	12/29
2.	1/50	7.	11/20
3.	1 1/4	8.	1 13/15
4.	9 3/7	9.	33
5.	14/15	10.	22/35

Working with Addition of Decimals

1.	6074.6132	7.	21.62
2.	142.205	8.	59.52
3.	1.988	9.	65.71
4.	1961.1713	10.	28.99
5.	56.97	11.	35.99
6.	70.8	12.	28.12

Working with Subtraction of Decimals

1.	321.0155	7.	423.697
2.	0.051	8.	66.8
3.	9012.333	9.	8703.8
4.	7049.263	10.	853.1
5.	7.977	11.	553.9
6.	601.05	12.	939.2

Working with Multiplication of Decimals

1.	75.28	7.	3.6888
2.	1.6168	8.	7.344
3.	336.742	9.	320.1
4.	78.0861	10.	0.2475
5.	0.102	11.	67.6208
6.	30.1515	12.	50.47

Working with Division of Decimals

1.	45	7.	48.1
2.	112	8.	83.4
3.	7.08	9.	46.7
4.	20.5	10.	0.0565
5.	0.05	11.	49.456
6.	401.2	12.	1.084

Working with Roman numerals

1.	VIISS	5.	CI
2.	XXXV	6.	XVSS
3.	XLI	7.	XCIX
4.	LXV	8.	MMV

Working with Roman numerals

1.	30	5.	150
2.	14	6.	95
3.	49	7.	75
4.	1 1/2	8.	2010

Module: METHODS OF CALCULATION

Working with Methods of Calculation

1.	2 tablets	13.	2.25 mL
2.	1 ½ tablets	14.	3.5 mL
3.	2 pills	15.	30 cc
4.	0.25 tablet	16.	0.6 mL
5.	3 caplets	17.	gr 1/75
6.	3.5 mL	18.	20 mL
7.	3 tablets	19.a.	0.4 mL
8.	0.5 mL	b.	5 doses
9.	3 mL	20.a.	0.8 mL
10.	16 mL	b.	5 doses
11.	10 days	c.	0.65 mL
12.	10 days	d.	6 doses

Module: SYSTEMS OF MEASUREMENT

Working with the Metric System

1.	3500 mL		11.	1000 mm
2.	700 mL		12.	1650 g
3.	1 g		13.	1.5 L
4.	0.1 mg		14.	2500 mg
5.	10,000 mcg		15.	0.75 g
6.	2000 mcg		16.	500 mg
7.	0.0356 g		17.	0.075 mg
8.	0.00745 L		18.	450 mcg
9.	0.007 dm		19.	1200 g
10.	10,000 M		20.	40 mm

Working with the Apothecaries' System

1. ℥ iii

2. ♏ x

3. ℥ viii

4. ♏ xiv

5. gr viiss

6. gr xxxiv

7. ℥ ss

8. ℥ xix

9. ℥ iv

10. ♏ xii

11.

12.

Working wth the Household System

1. 6 tsp
2. 2 T
3. 3 tsp
4. 16 oz
5. 8 oz
6. 6 tsp
7. 1 T

8. 10 mL

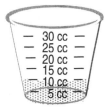

9. 24 oz
10. 8 oz

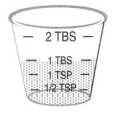

Working with Conversions between Systems

1. 15 mL
2. 0.4 mg
3. 1 oz
4. gr 0.005
5. 180 mg
6. 30 mg

7. ℥ iss

8. ℥ iii

9. 0.6 mg
10. gtt iv

11. 4 t
12. 9 t
13. 480 cc
14. 2.54 cm
15. gr xv
16. 165 lb
17. 90 kg
18. 3 cc
19. ½ tablet
20. 360 cc
21. 184.8 lb
22. 2 tablets
23. 0.33 mL

Module: INTAKE AND OUTPUT

Working with Intake and Output

1.   I 960 cc
     O 440 cc

2.   I 270 cc
     O 280 cc

3.   O 1410 cc

4.   I 300 cc
     O 270 cc

5.   I 2020 cc
     O 595 cc

6.   I 1000 cc

7.   I 1274 cc
     O 425 cc

8.   I 1330 cc
     O 605 cc

9.   I 970 cc
     O 480 cc

10. I 675 cc

Working with Nasogastric Tube Feeding Problems

1. 80 mL
2. 466 cc
3. 119 mL
4. 750 cc
5. 237 mL
6. 711 mL
7. 200 mL

Module: READING MEDICATION LABELS

Working with Reading Medication Labels

1.   a Mirapex
     b. pramipexole dihydrochloride

c. 0.25 mg/tablet
d. Tablet
e. Oral

2.   a. fentanyl citrate
b. 250 mcg/5mL
c. Milliliters
d. IV or IM
e. Yes
f. Single dose
g. 3 mL

3.   a. Cipro
b. ciprofloxacin
c. Dilute with 100 to 200 mL of suitable diluent

4.   a. morphine sulfate
b. 15 mg/mL
c. 20 mL
d. SC, IM, or IV
e. Yes
f. No
g. 0.67 mL

5.   a. 10 mL

6.   a. diazepam
b. 5 mg/mL
c. IM or IV
d. Yes
e. No
f. 2.5 mL

7. a. Lovenox
    b. 30 mg/0.3 mL
    c. SC
    d. Store at room temperature

8. a. meperidine HCl
    b. 75 mg/mL
    c. IM, SC, or IV
    d. Yes
    e. 0.8 mL

9. a. NPH Iletin II
    b. Purified Pork

10. a. Humalog
    b. 6 U

11. a. Novolin 70/30
    b. 22 U

12. Humulin 50/50

Module: ADMINISTRATION OF ORAL MEDICATIONS

Working with Administration of Oral Medications

1. 2 tablets
2. 2 tablets
3. 1 tablet

4. 1/2 tablet
5. 2 tablets
6. 960 mg

7.	8 mL	14.	1/2 tablet
8.	1 tsp	15.	1 tablet
9.	20 mL	16.	2 tablets
10.	1 tablet	17.	20 mL
11.	10 mL	18.	10 mL
12.	2 tablets	19.	720 mg
13.	5 days	20.	1 tablet

Module: SYRINGES AND NEEDLES

Working with Syringes

1. 0.3 mL

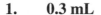

2. 0.66 mL

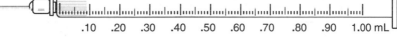

3. 0.09 mL

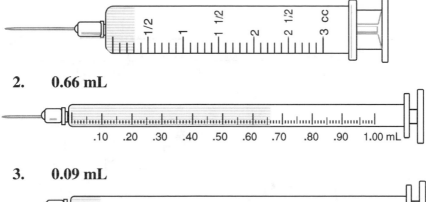

4. ℳ viiss

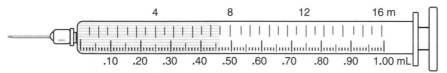

5. ♏ xv

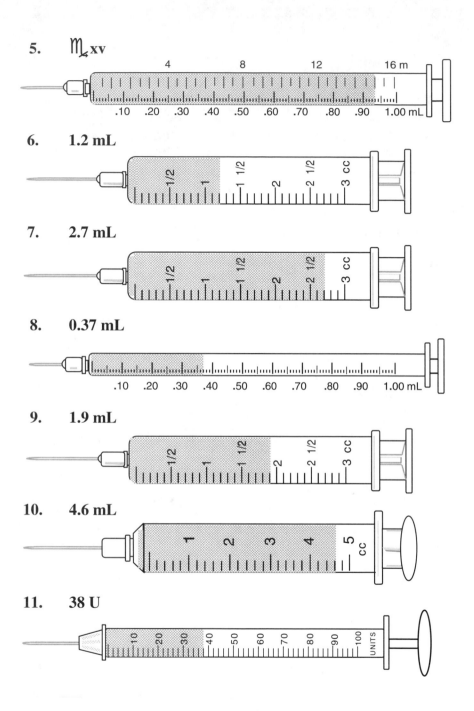

6. 1.2 mL

7. 2.7 mL

8. 0.37 mL

9. 1.9 mL

10. 4.6 mL

11. 38 U

12. 27 U

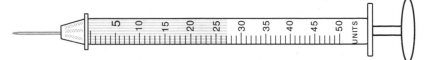

13. 7 U

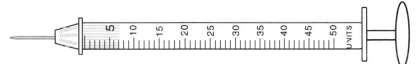

14. 7 U

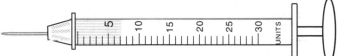

15. 16 U

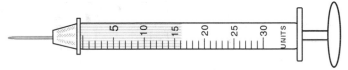

16. 56 U

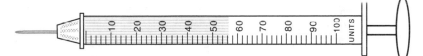

17. 3.8 mL

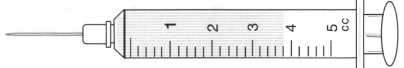

Working with Needles

1.   28G 1/2 ”
2.   21–23G 1 ½”
3.   26–27G 3/8”
4.   21–23G 2”
5.   25G 5/8”
6.   18–19G 1”

Working with Syringes and Needles

1.   **Meperidine 75 mg (1 mL) IM**

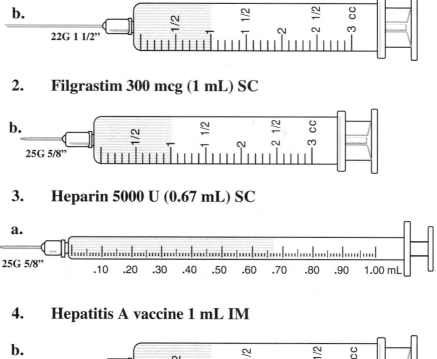

b.

22G 1 1/2”

2.   **Filgrastim 300 mcg (1 mL) SC**

b.

25G 5/8”

3.   **Heparin 5000 U (0.67 mL) SC**

a.

25G 5/8”

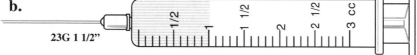

.10 .20 .30 .40 .50 .60 .70 .80 .90 1.00 mL

4.   **Hepatitis A vaccine 1 mL IM**

b.

23G 1 1/2”

5. **Ketorolac 60 mg (2 mL) IM**

b.

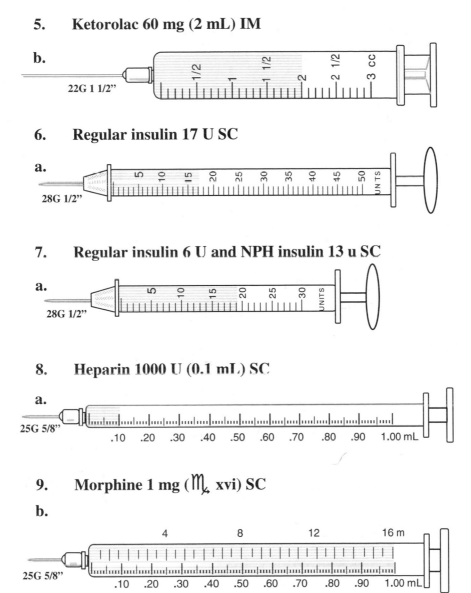

6. **Regular insulin 17 U SC**

a.

7. **Regular insulin 6 U and NPH insulin 13 u SC**

a.

8. **Heparin 1000 U (0.1 mL) SC**

a.

9. **Morphine 1 mg (♏ xvi) SC**

b.

Module: ADMINISTRATION OF PARENTERAL MEDICATIONS

Working with Administration of Parenteral Medications

1. 0.2 mL
2. 1.5 mL
3. 0.25 mL
4. 2 mL

Fill in the syringe.

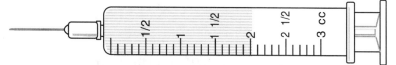

5. meperidine HCl = 0.6 mL
   glycopyrrolate = 0.4 mL

   Total amount   = 1 mL
   Fill in the syringe with the total amount.

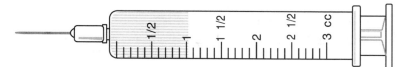

6. 0.1 mL
   Fill in the syringe.

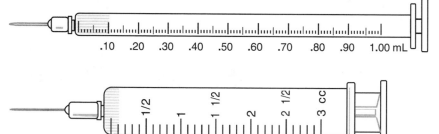

7.   0.4 mL

8.   16 minims

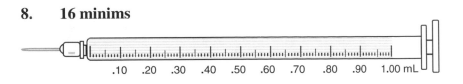

.10   .20   .30   .40   .50   .60   .70   .80   .90   1.00 mL

9.   0.6 mL
Fill in the ordered dose in each syringe.

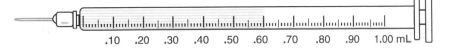

.10   .20   .30   .40   .50   .60   .70   .80   .90   1.00 mL

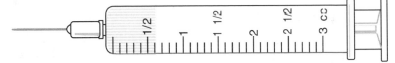

10.   0.25 mL
Fill in the syringe.

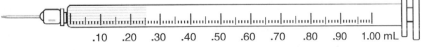

.10   .20   .30   .40   .50   .60   .70   .80   .90   1.00 mL

11.   2.5 mL

12.   23 U
Fill in the syringe.

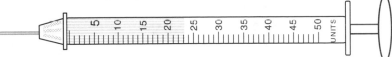

13.   52 U
Fill in the syringe.

14. **21 U**
Fill in the syringe.

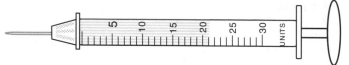

15. **19 U**
Fill in the syringe.

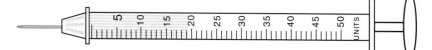

16. **2 U**
Fill in the syringe.

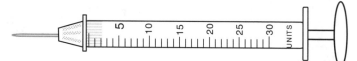

17. **29 U**
Fill in the syringe.

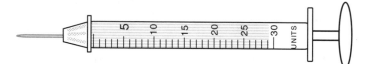

Module: RECONSTITUTION OF POWDERED MEDICATIONS

Working with Single-Strength Reconstitution

1.a. **2.5 mL**
  b. **Sterile water for injection**
  c. **330 mg/mL**

1.d. 0.76 mL
2.a. 4.6 mL
  b. Bacteriostatic water for injection
  c. 200,000 units/mL
  d. 1.5 mL
3. Date and time of reconstitution; nurse's initials
4.a. 2 mL
  b. Sterile water for injection
  c. 125 mg/mL
  d. 1.6 mL
5.a. 1 g/2.6 mL
  b. 1.3 mL
6.a. 5.7 mL
  b. Sterile water for injection
  c. 250 mg/1.5 mL
  d. 2.7 mL
7.a. 87 mL
  b. 250 mg/5 mL
  c. 10 mL
8. Date and time of reconstitution; nurse's initials

Working with Multiple-Strength Reconstitution

1. The smallest volume of diluent
2.a. 100 mg/mL
  b. 7.5 mL
  c. Date and time of reconstitution; nurse's initials;
     circle selected volume of diluent and
     corresponding dosage strength.
3.a. 100,000 units/mL
  b. 500,000 units/mL
  c. 9.6 mL of diluent – give 10 mL
     4.6 mL of diluent – give 5 mL
     1.6 mL of diluent – give 2 mL

4.a. 75 mL of diluent – 250,000 units/mL
33 mL of diluent – 500,000 units/mL
11.5 mL of diluent – 1,000,000 units/mL

  b. 75 mL of diluent – give 3 mL
33 mL of diluent – give 1.5 mL
11.5 mL of diluent – give 0.75 mL

  c. 7 days

  d. Date and time of reconstitution; nurse's initials; circle selected volume of diluent and corresponding dosage strength.

5.a. 3.5 mL of diluent – 500 mg/mL
7.2 mL of diluent – 250 mg/mL

  b. 3.5 mL of diluent – give 1.4 mL
7.2 mL of diluent – give 2.8 mL

  c. 1 hour at room temperature; 6 hours under refrigeration.

  d. 3.5 mL is preferable so that the volume of the IM injection is smaller.

  e. Date and time of reconstitution; nurse's initials; circle selected volume of diluent and the corresponding dosage strength.

Module: IV CALCULATIONS

Working with Milliliters per Hour

1. 83 cc/hr
2. 63 cc/hr
3. 125 mL/hr
4. 167 mL/hr
5. 100 mL/hr
6. 167 mL/hr
7. 50 mL/hr

Working with Flow Rate

1. 125 gtt/min
2. 21 gtt/min
3. 21 gtt/min
4. 8 gtt/min
5. 11 gtt/min
6. 33 gtt/min

Working with IV Push Medications

1. 4 – 5 minutes
2. 6 – 10 minutes
3. 1 – 2 minutes
4. 2 – 3 minutes
5. 2 minutes
6. 1 minute
7. 2 minutes or longer (3 minutes or 8–15 minutes)

Working with Infusion Time

1. 8 hours
2. 8 hours 20 minutes
3. 13 hours 20 minutes
4. 6 hours 24 minutes
5. 30 minutes
6. 3 hours 20 minutes

Working with Completion Time

1. 4:00 PM or 1600
2. 6:10 PM or 1810
3. 6:00 AM or 0600
4. 3:30 AM or 0330
5. 8:45 PM or 2045
6. 2:00 PM or 1400

Working with Infusion and Completion Time

1. **Infusion Time = 9 hours**
   Completion Time = 8:00 PM or 2000
2. **Infusion Time = 3 hours 30 minutes**
   Completion Time = 7:00 PM or 1900
3. **Infusion Time = 5 hours**
   Completion Time = 1:00 AM or 0100
4. **Infusion Time = 4 hours 40 minutes**
   Completion Time = 11:40 AM or 1140
5. **Infusion Time = 5 hours**
   Completion Time = 2:00 AM or 0200

Labeling IV Bags

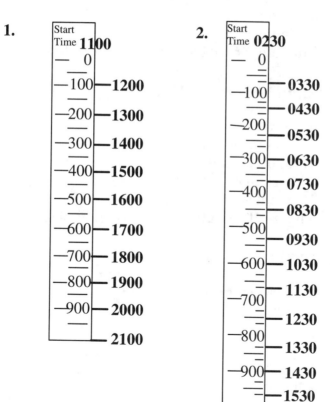

1.

Start Time **1100**
— 0
—100 —**1200**
—200 —**1300**
—300 —**1400**
—400 —**1500**
—500 —**1600**
—600 —**1700**
—700 —**1800**
—800 —**1900**
—900 —**2000**
—**2100**

2.

Start Time **0230**
— 0
—100 —**0330**
—**0430**
—200 —**0530**
—300 —**0630**
—**0730**
—400 —**0830**
—500 —**0930**
—600 —**1030**
—**1130**
—700 —**1230**
—800 —**1330**
—900 —**1430**
—**1530**
1550

3.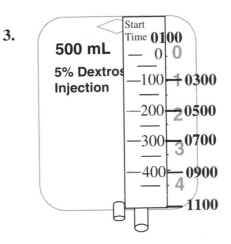

500 mL

5% Dextros
Injection

Start Time 0100

— 0 | 0
—100 0300
—200 0500
—300 0700
—400 0900
1100

4.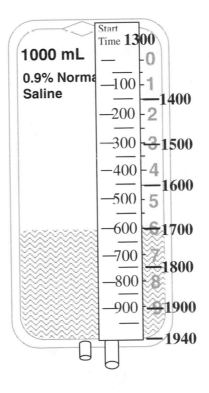

1000 mL

0.9% Norm
Saline

Start Time 1300

— 0
—100 1
—200 2 1400
—300 3 1500
—400 4
—500 5 1600
—600 6 1700
—700 7
—800 8 1800
—900 9 1900
1940

5.

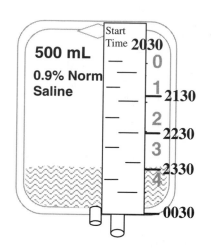

Module: PEDIATRIC CALCULATIONS

Working with Administering Medications to Children

1.   **2 tablets**
2.   **14 mL**
3.   **3 tablets**
4.   **2 tablets**
5.a. **2.5 mL**
  b.

6.a. **0.16 mL**
  b.

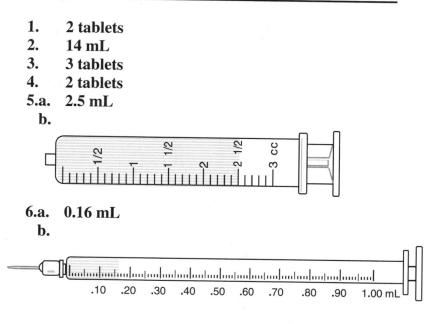

7.a. 1.2 mL
   b. 60 mL/hr
8.a. 100 gtt/min
   b. 1430

Dosage Based on Body Weight

1.a. 210 mg q.12h.
   b. Yes, the dose is safe.
2.a. 400 mcg/dose
   b. Yes, the dose is safe.
3.a. 180 mg/day
   b. Yes, the dose is safe.
4.a. 10.5 mg q.3–4h.
   b. No, the dose is not safe.
5.a. 258.5 mg
   b. No, the dose is not safe.

Dosage Based on Body Surface Area

1.a. 5.6 mg q.6h.
   b. Yes, the dose is safe.
2.a. 198 mg/dose
   b. No, the dose is not safe.
3.a. 8.625 mg/q.1–2 weeks up to 12 weeks.
   b. No, the dose is not safe.
4.a. 0.22 mg/day
   b. Yes, the dose is safe.
5.a. 590 mg q.8h. for 7 days
   b. Yes, the dose is safe.

Working with Nastrogastric Fluid Replacement

1.a. 100 mL/hr
  b. 150 mL/hr
  c. 7 hours 36 minutes
  d. 2236 or 10:36 PM
2.a. 63 mL/hr
  b. 22 mL/hr
  c. 3 hours
  d. 1500 or 3:00 PM
3.a. 4 hours
  b. 0830 or 8:30 AM
4.a. 4 hours 30 minutes
  b. 0315 or 3:15 AM

Module: TITRATION OF IV MEDICATIONS

Solving Titration Problems

1.a. 6 mg/hr
  b. 6 mL/hr
  c. No
2.a. 60 mg/hr
  b. 15 mL/hr
  c. 30 mL
3.a. 120 mL/hr
  b. 60 mL/hr
4. 20 mL/hr
5. 10 mL/hr
6. 68 mL/hr
7. 60 mg/hr
8. 100 mg/hr
9. 4 mg/min

10. 35 mL/hr
11. 56 mL/hr
12. 3 mL/hr
13. 38 mL/hr
14. 30 mL/hr
15. 120 mL/hr
16. 12 mL/hr
17. 6 mL/hr
18. 33 mL/hr
19.a. 55 mL/hr
  b. 66 mL/hr
20.a. Yes
  b. 51 mL/hr

Appendix

Body Surface Area Nomograms for Children

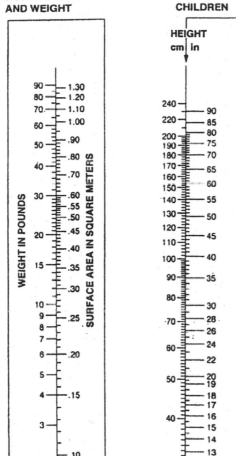

FOR CHILDREN OF NORMAL HEIGHT AND WEIGHT

NOMOGRAM FOR OTHER CHILDREN

(From Nelson Textbook of Pediatrics, ed 16. WB Saunders Co, Philadelphia, PA, 2000.)